The Healthy Baby Book

A Parent's Guide to
Preventing Birth Defects and Other
Long-Term Medical Problems Before,
During, and After Pregnancy

CAROLYN REUBEN

Foreword by Sumner J. Yaffe, M.D.

JEREMY P. TARCHER/PERIGEE

Jeremy P. Tarcher/Perigee Books
are published by
The Putnam Publishing Group
200 Madison Avenue
New York, NY 10016

Reader Please Note: This material has been collected and published for educational purposes only. It should not be used as a substitute for advice from your personal physician or specialists in the fields of genetics, pediatrics, and obstetrics.

Ideally, you will seek out and work with an environmentally aware and nutritionally knowledgeable practitioner who can guide you with personal attention to your individual situation.

The author and publisher offer this guidebook with the expectation that readers use the information contained within it at their own risk, and with the full knowledge that even if every single suggestion is followed to the letter, it is still possible to give birth to a child with a birth defect or long-range medical problem. The author and publisher, therefore, are not responsible for any adverse effects or consequences resulting from the use of this book. Please do not use the material presented here, if you are not willing to assume that risk.

Library of Congress Cataloging-in-Publication Data

Reuben, Carolyn, date
    The healthy baby book: a parent's guide to preventing birth defects and
other long-term medical problems before, during, and after pregnancy / Carolyn
Reuben : foreword by Sumner J. Yaffe.

        p.   cm.
    Includes bibliographical references and index.
    ISBN 0-87477-679-1
    1. Abnormalities, Human—Popular works.   2. Abnormalities, Human—
Prevention.   3. Abnormalities, Human—Etiology.   I. Title.
    RG626.R497   1992   92-23663 CIP
    618.3 ' 2—dc20

Jeremy P. Tarcher, Inc.
5858 Wilshire Blvd., Suite 200
Los Angeles, Calif. 90036

Published simultaneously in Canada

Design by Lee Fukui

Front cover photograph by Jerry Atnip/Superstock

Manufactured in the United States of America
10   9   8   7   6   5   4   3   2   1

This book is printed on acid-free paper.

For Natanya,
whose name means gift from God,

and for all the world's children,
who are gifts, too.

Contents

Acknowledgments   x

Preface   xii

Foreword   xvii

Introduction   1
    The Definition of Birth Defects   2
    The Incidence of Birth Defects   2
    Who's at Risk   4
    The Causes of Birth Defects   5
    Genetics and Birth Defects   5
    The Environment and Birth Defects   12
    Prenatal Testing for Birth Defects   16

PART ONE: BEFORE PREGNANCY   21

Preconception Care   23

Pre-existing Medical Conditions   27
    AIDS   27
    Diabetes   28
    Epilepsy   32

Occupational Hazards for Women   34
    The Woman Working at Home   37

The Father's Role   39

    Age and Inheritance   39
    Environmental Influences on Sperm   40

PART TWO: DURING PREGNANCY   47

Prenatal Care   49

Prematurity, Low Birth Weight, and Stress   52

    Stress Reduction   53
    The French Model   54

Diet and Nutrition   58

    Nutritional Deficiencies and Birth Defects 58
    A Note About Dieting During Pregnancy   63

Prescription and Over-the-Counter Drugs   65

    Over-the-Counter Drugs   70

Recreational Drugs   75

    Alcohol   75
    Coffee and Tea   77
    LSD, Marijuana, Heroin, and Cocaine   78
    Nicotine   80

Environmental Toxicants   83

    Air   83
    Water   87
    Hidden Contamination   91
    Electromagnetic Radiation   93
    Pesticides   99

Exercise   101

Gestational Diabetes   105

Infectious Diseases   108

    Chicken Pox (Varicella)   108
    Cytomegalovirus (CMV)   110
    Fifth Disease   111

German Measles (Rubella)   112
Hepatitis B   113
Herpes Simplex   114
Syphilis   117
Toxoplasmosis   118

Labor and Delivery   120

Incompatible Blood Type   120
Fetal Monitoring   121
Drugs During Labor   123
Cesarean Section   124

PART THREE: AFTER PREGNANCY   129

Infant Feeding   131

The Breast-Fed Baby   131
The Formula-Fed Baby   136

Sudden Infant Death Syndrome   141

Your Child's Environment   144

Lead and Other Heavy Metals   144
Radiation   146
Cigarettes   147
Chemicals and Pesticides   147

Afterword   151

Appendix A: The Most Common Birth Defects   153

Appendix B: Resources   160

Hotlines   160
Associations   163
Resources for a Safe Home Environment   164
Books   164

Glossary   166

Select Bibliography   168

Index   181

Acknowledgments

The following experts consented to be interviewed at length, made sure I had the materials I needed, or read and critiqued the section of my manuscript that related to their area of expertise. Although I am responsible for whatever mistakes there may be, the richness of detail is due to the yeoman's effort of all mentioned below to share their time and wisdom. Thanks . . .

To the March of Dimes Director of Science Information: Richard Leavitt.

To those from the Environmental Protection Agency: Michael Bandrowski; Michael Berry, Ph.D.; Gerald Chernoff, Ph.D.; Michael Davis, Ph.D.; Robert Elias, Ph.D.; William Ewald; Bruce Henschel; Patrick Kennedy; Carole Kimmel, Ph.D.; Gary Kimmel, Ph.D.; Bruce Macler, Ph.D.; Shelly Rosenblum; Sherry Selevan, Ph.D.; Chon Shoaf, Ph.D.; Lance Wallace, Ph.D.; and Marie Pfaff.

To those now or formerly from the Centers for Disease Control: Susan Chu, Ph.D.; José Cordero, M.D.; Solomon Iyasu, M.D.; Charles LeBaron, M.D.; Michele Lynberg, Ph.D.; David Nelson, M.D., M.P.H.; Gregg Sylvester, M.D., M.P.H.; and Thomas Torok, M.D.

To those in academia and research: Bruce Beckwith, M.D.; Cheston Berlin Jr., M.D.; Eric Block, Ph.D.; James Clapp III, M.D.; Christine Dunkel-Schetter, Ph.D.; Dale Hattis, Ph.D.; John Kitzmiller, M.D.; Marci Lobel, Ph.D.; Donald Mattison, M.D.; Lewis Mehl, M.D., Ph.D.; Merry-K. Moos, F.N.P., M.P.H.; Andrew Olshan, Ph.D.; Gayle Peterson, LCSW, Ph.D.; Lois Jovanovic Peterson, M.D.; Frances Tennant, M.D.; James Warram, M.D.; and Barry Zuckerman, M.D.

To those from the State of California Department of Health Services: Ray Neutra, M.D.; Ronald Roberto, M.D.; and Alexis Milea.

To those professionals with particular expertise: Belinda Barnes; Susan Brandle, IBCLC (lactation consultant); Troy Brannan; Harold Buttram, M.D.; Jack DeMarco; Don Deno, Ph.D.; Karen Evon, IBCLC (lactation consultant); Judy Flanagan CNM (midwife); Paul Fleiss, M.D.; Nancy Goldman, M.D.; Richard Gould, M.D.; Robert Frantz, M.D.; Perry Gottesfeld; Arthur Grix, M.D.; Nadia Henry; Maria Iorillo; Erik Jansson; Nadine Joseph; Nan Koehler; Richard Kunin, M.D.; Fred Lerner, D.C., Ph.D.; Linda Marcuz, R.N.; Neil Massoud, Pharm.D.; Betty Mekdeci; Beth Moser, R.N.; Egan O'Connor; Judy Polkow; Jeanne Rose; Cappy Rothman, M.D.; Wallace Sampson, M.D.; Jim Shultz; Joan Scott; Patricia Simmons, M.D.; Leon Sternfeld, M.D.; Liz Stierman; Jack Thrasher, Ph.D.; John Williams III, M.D.; Marilyn Wind, Ph.D.; and William Wolverton, Ph.D.

To those who assisted my collection of medical research: Carlson Health Sciences Library staff (UC Davis); Kathy Kneer (California Birth Defects Monitoring Program); Mary Ann Mahoney (California Occupational and Environmental Health Library); Dorothy Thurmond (Guttman Library, Sacramento-El Dorado Medical Society); Maureen Sanderson (National Center for Health Statistics); UC Davis Medical Center (Sacramento) library staff; the American College of Obstetricians and Gynecologists; and the American Academy of Pediatrics.

To those involved in publishing the manuscript: My agent Barbara Lowenstein, who has a happy client; my publisher Jeremy Tarcher, who entrusted his idea to me; my in-house editor Rick Benzel, whose talent transformed excessive pages into a concise handbook; editor Mary Ellen Strote, who released the chaff and refined the kernel; Jennifer Boynton, who kept an expert eye on production; and Sue Lowe, copy editor par excellence.

To my parents, whose support and love was ever-present: Betty and Jack Reuben.

Preface

Having gone through my only pregnancy when I was thirty-eight years old, I know firsthand how scary ordinary activities can become when you are worried about the well-being of your developing child. I am talking about everyday activities, such as cleaning house, drinking a glass of wine, or taking over-the-counter medication. Simply being pregnant can be scary if you happen to be an older mom.

We all tend to avoid discomfort and find subjects such as birth defects difficult to face. Nevertheless, by facing this issue, a woman can do much to improve the outcome of her pregnancy. By sharing with you what I've learned about preventable dangers that might lead to birth defects, I hope to help you protect your child from harm before, during, and even after pregnancy.

Although the term *birth defects* is convenient shorthand for a book title, it does not communicate the breadth of issues presented in this book. We generally imagine physical disabilities when we hear the term *birth defects*, but very few of the babies born each year have obvious malformations, such as a cleft lip or missing limb. Thus I discuss the prevention of not only physical defects but also spontaneous abortions, miscarriages, and stillbirths, as well as premature birth and low birth weight, which account for significant health problems and financial burdens. I also address that thirty years of research studies have linked a parent's exposure to medications, illegal drugs, chemicals, and infections to problems their offspring may have with thinking and behavior years after birth—in childhood and adulthood.

A NOTE ABOUT TERMINOLOGY

We often believe that what we say is shaped by external reality. Actually, instead, words do much of the shaping by creating the context in which we look at our world and the people in it. In writing this book, I have had to recognize and change a number of my own habits of terminology that created an inappropriate and sometimes unkind picture of reality. The following is an explanation of a few choices I have made regarding word usage.

Since about half of the population are "he" and half are "she," I have chosen to assign gender randomly throughout the text.

In spite of the fact that trisomy 21 is often called Down's syndrome in the medical literature, I use the term *Down syndrome*. In 1975 an international group of advisers recommended to the National Institutes of Health that whenever the name of a medical condition refers to the physician or scientist who named it (for example, J. Langdon Down, a nineteenth-century British physician), the possessive should not be used. The NIH rule for nomenclature is followed in this book.

I also follow most of the guidelines advocated by the Research and Training Center on Independent Living, in Lawrence, Kansas. These include focusing on the human being rather than the person's medical condition when writing about people who have disabilities. For example, the guidelines stress that it is unnecessarily sensationalizing to say someone suffers from, is afflicted with, or is the victim of a condition.

I have also chosen to say, for example, "a boy with epilepsy" (not, an epileptic); "a child with spastic muscles" (not, a spastic); and "a woman with diabetes" (not, a diabetic)—since people are more than their medical condition.

The power of language to alter our sense of reality is elementary yet profound, and consciously controlling our language is a simple way for us to help create a humane, loving world.

HOW THE BOOK IS ORGANIZED

In the first chapter, I provide an overview of birth defects and an expanded definition of the topic. I include an examination of the incidence of birth defects, who is at risk, the difference between defects caused by genetics and those caused by other factors, and the testing procedures available to parents to detect problems before or during pregnancy. This is important background information that includes references to the science of genetics. I hope I have succeeded in writing it so that even the technical material is clear to most parents.

The remainder of the book describes the most serious hazards to the health of your baby and offers specific steps you can take to eliminate or diminish your risks before, during, and after pregnancy.

I have written this book for every mother- and father-to-be and for those with newborns. If you are about to embark on parenthood, you are in the best position to prevent birth defects. You have time to prepare your body, to reduce exposure to toxic substances and infections, and to improve your diet before the blossom of your efforts—that beautiful son or daughter—makes an appearance. If you are already pregnant, you will learn how improvements in your daily nutrition, work environment, drug usage, and emotional stress level will greatly benefit the developing baby. If you have just given birth, you will be interested in learning how breast milk and various formulas can influence your baby's health, what you might do to prevent sudden infant death syndrome, and how to avoid environmental dangers.

This book also reveals the economic consequences to our nation of ignoring preconception and prenatal care. One of the most surprising facts that I learned from the research for this book is that birth defects can be a link between the boardroom and the bedroom (or, some may say, the kitchen). Here is an example: Imagine a lake into which company "X" has dumped industrial waste. Over time, mercury compounds in the waste are chemically altered by acid rain and turn into a toxic form that rises up the food chain from plankton to fish. Humans then eat the polluted fish, influencing the health of unborn children exposed to the toxins through their mother's diet.

Once we discover such close connections between business, the environment, and reproductive health, we must be unafraid to insist on safety—even at the cost of inconvenience. We must remind everyone—employers, legislators, educators, and government authorities—that a child with birth defects is not only a family issue but also a nationwide responsibility influencing our society's medical, mental health, and educational institutions. In fact, the March of Dimes estimates that birth defects cost America billions of dollars a year in increased medical expenses.

The information in this book came from many sources. I interviewed experts, searched through medical studies published in the United States and Europe, and read books and transcripts of the proceedings of international academic symposia. As in all branches of modern medicine, new research in this field appears continually, but at some point I had to stop collecting data to publish what I'd learned so you could put it to good use. Although most of my suggestions are based on thoroughly documented discoveries, some are still controversial. How many and which ones you choose to act upon will be a very personal decision.

No matter how conscientiously one follows the steps suggested in this book, there is always the possibility of a birth defect. Although we are partners in the act of creating this universe with the unseen force that guides it, neither we nor our doctors are omnipotent beings. So, as we endeavor to do all that we can to have a perfect child, we must be ready to admit that we can act only according to the knowledge, time, and resources available to us. Having done that, we may be able to release ourselves from the self-defeating stranglehold of guilt.

In spite of prenatal exposure to drugs, pesticides, background radiation, and many other dangers of our modern world, most babies are born healthy and develop normally. Yet, why ignore what information does exist that you, as concerned parents, can put to good use? I hope my efforts, coupled with your own, help you achieve the healthy child you desire.

Carolyn Reuben
Sacramento, California

Foreword

For thirty years I have been looking for a book like the one you hold in your hands. I have been in the field of pediatric pharmacology, studying the effects of drugs on fetuses, babies, and children, that long. And throughout my career I've wished to be able to hand parents-to-be a book containing the quantity and quality of practical advice found in this one.

I especially like the fact that Carolyn Reuben expands the definition of birth defects beyond physical malformations apparent at birth. Almost a generation has passed since the DES debacle of the 1970s, when teenagers and women in their twenties were found to have developed vaginal cancer due to their exposure to the drug DES (diethylstilbestrol) before birth. The causal relationship between fetal exposure to certain drugs and alterations in brain function that may not be apparent until the child starts school is difficult to establish. By that time, the parent, teacher, pediatrician, or child development specialist may blame any number of causes other than prenatal drug exposure for a lowered IQ or learning disability. For moral and ethical reasons, human experiments to prove the long-term effect of pharmaceuticals during pregnancy and delivery cannot be done. Scientists have to work on animals, as I did with phenobarbital.

Phenobarbital is the most widely prescribed drug worldwide, used both within multi-ingredient formulas to alleviate anxiety, and given on its own, as in cases of epilepsy. In an experiment that I and a colleague performed years ago, we found only a third of mature female rats who had been exposed to phenobarbital prenatally had normal menstrual cycles. About two-thirds of the females were infertile. Male rats exposed to the drug were more likely to be infertile than unexposed animals, and had half the level of the male hormone, testosterone. Can we extrapolate these findings to humans? Scientifically we can't, but the striking functional abnormalities in the animals give us some concern.

What I do know is that about one in five married couples in the United States is currently experiencing some degree of infertility, and the incidence of this problem has increased by 50 percent within the last couple decades. I know that we in America spend a higher portion of our gross national product on health care than any other nation on earth, yet we are an embarrassing 23rd in the world in infant mortality. I know that one in twelve infants born alive has an obvious congenital defect visible during the first year of life, and 16 percent of the population have birth defects that appear as children mature. I know that school test scores across America are not encouraging, and that each year it seems more common to hear diagnoses like "Attention Deficit Disorder" and "Learning Disabled" to describe school children.

I also know it's true that most drugs cross the placenta and that, with rare exception, there is no barrier. Consequently, although we have not experienced a second thalidomide-like disaster of severely malformed newborns, we must not be complacent, because there is plenty of evidence for the hypothesis that we are being affected by the sea of drugs in which we live.

Unfortunately, studies of drug use during pregnancy show women taking at least four, and sometimes many more, prescribed drugs (in Texas, women in one study took from three to twenty-nine drugs, including prescription and over-the-counter remedies, during a pregnancy)! If you look at a computerized payment system like Medicaid and track the drug prescriptions of women, you'll suddenly see a big blip indicating an increase in the number of drugs prescribed, and you'll know that this is when particular women became pregnant!

Another reason for my enthusiasm about this particular book is its discussion of preconceptual care. If we as individuals and as a nation are really going to move in the area of having every baby be born wanted and healthy and reduce both infant mortality and congenital malformations, we ought to plan for that baby before it is conceived. After all, a farmer wouldn't think of throwing seeds into an unprepared soil. Human fetuses are highly susceptible to damage soon after conception. So why do we think that the appropriate order of human reproduction is to wait for a positive pregnancy test and only then try to stop smoking, refuse the same margarita freely downed the day before, and shove deeper under the sink the toxic cleaning solvents that yesterday were used to scour the stove? How much more logical and useful to put away the cigarettes, alcohol, chemicals, and pharmaceuticals months, or at least weeks, before new life begins.

Think about it this way: Thalidomide did not happen to pregnant women. Pregnancy happened to women who were taking thalidomide for nervousness or as a nighttime sedative.

Pregnancy is a symptom-producing event! A pregnant woman is often nauseous at the beginning of pregnancy and has swollen feet and legs plus digestive disturbances nearer to delivery. That doesn't mean if you are pregnant you have to take a pharmaceutical to treat every symptom. In fact, in this book you will learn about a greater number of nontoxic, non-pharmaceutical solutions to common medical problems.

I challenge physicians to be more conservative in prescribing for pregnant women. I urge medical professionals as well as women and men en route to parenthood to read this book with care. There is much more in here than the danger of medications and environmental chemicals. You'll find something worth remembering regardless of what stage of parenthood you are in: preconception, pregnant, or coping with weighty responsibilities after delivery. At the very least, you'll approach your obstetrician or pediatrician a better informed medical consumer, which is exactly why this is the practical guide I hoped someday would find its way into your hands.

Sumner J. Yaffe, M.D.
Director, Center for Research
for Mothers and Children
National Institute of Child Health
and Human Development
National Institutes of Health
Bethesda, Maryland

Introduction

From the dawn of human history pregnant women and fathers-to-be, eagerly looking forward to the birth of healthy children, often attempted to ensure this happy outcome by using ritual, prayer, or other supplications to the spiritual world. Until quite recently, our own culture has not been much more educated about the causes of birth defects. Western medicine discounted the power of evil spirits but, having few other explanations for the presence of birth defects, often simply blamed chance.

Until the middle of this century, most doctors believed that the womb was a stress-free, unsullied environment, a soft barricade that protected an unborn child from harm. It took an observant Australian doctor to notice, just fifty years ago, that patients who contracted German measles (rubella) during their first trimester of pregnancy frequently gave birth to babies with certain specific defects relating to the heart, eyes, and ears. A few years later, the atom bombs dropped on Hiroshima and Nagasaki proved that radiation, too, could be a potent cause of birth defects, including small brains and mental retardation.

Then, beginning in 1959, people around the world were shocked by evidence that the tranquilizer and antinausea drug thalidomide caused severe limb and organ abnormalities when taken by a pregnant woman from the 20th to 36th day after conception.

We now know that infectious diseases, environmental agents, and pharmaceuticals can cross the rich network of blood vessels that form the placenta and may influence the developing fetus. We also know that even long before pregnancy begins, both the egg and the sperm can be affected by the parents' nutrition and exposure to chemicals, radiation, and other environmental factors.

At first glance, our influence on the health of an unborn baby may seem to be a frightening and overwhelming responsibility. It can, however, provide us comfort and power, for it means that unlike peoples of past centuries, we are not helpless victims of evil spirits or chance. We can use our newfound knowledge to plan for, create, and nurture our offspring with greater confidence than ever before.

THE DEFINITION OF BIRTH DEFECTS

In this book I define the term *birth defect* in its broadest sense. I include any structural, functional, or metabolic abnormality, disease, or disadvantageous mental, emotional, or behavioral characteristic that results from circumstances before, around, or following the time of conception, development, or birth.

Most people consider a birth defect to be any structural malformation or disease, evident at the moment of birth, that has major cosmetic or medical significance for the newborn. By school age, however, a perfectly formed and disease-free child who was exposed in the womb to certain pharmaceuticals or street drugs may exhibit abnormal behavior or learning disabilities that are specifically due to prenatal exposure to mind-damaging substances. Some schoolage children who were born prematurely or weighed less than five and a half pounds after nine months in the womb may also have emotional and physical problems. Although such symptoms may be hidden for years, they are nonetheless often evidence of a birth defect. Juvenile diabetes and a high susceptibility to cancer are now counted among the serious birth defects that may not appear until years or even decades after birth.

THE INCIDENCE OF BIRTH DEFECTS

There are nearly 4 million babies born each year in America, but exactly how many are born with birth defects is difficult to say. No national policy standardizes the way that birth defects are defined or recorded; some states compile detailed birth registries, but their reports vary widely in accuracy.

Different estimates offer us different perspectives on the incidence of structural birth defects. The most inclusive estimate is given by the March of Dimes, which suggests that about 7 percent of all Americans have some form of significant birth defect, including genetically determined degenerative diseases that appear in later life. The Centers for Disease Control (CDC) estimate that 2 to 3 percent (around 280,000) of American infants are born with serious or disabling malformations each year. A study by other researchers of more than 50,000 deliveries in twelve American institutions concluded that more than 15 percent of all one-year-olds had some sort of physical abnormality. (This figure, however, includes even minor abnormalities, such as birthmarks, which were not included in the other surveys.)

Nearly a third of the population of children in hospital wards are there due to birth defects. Moreover, according to the CDC, the combination of birth defects, premature birth, and sudden infant death syndrome accounts for more than 50 percent of all infant deaths each year. According to the March of Dimes, about 40,000 infants die before their first birthday, and one in five of those deaths is due to birth defects.

Perhaps the most significant statistic, however, is the incidence of specific birth defects. When the CDC investigated 38 structural malformations, they found that 29 malformations seemed to be increasing, particularly heart defects, missing or malformed kidneys, and gastroschisis, a rare abnormality of the abdominal wall. See Table 1 for an abbreviated list of birth defects and their incidence; you can find a more comprehensive list of specific birth defects in Appendix A.

Table 1. Prevalence of a few common birth defects

Birth Defect	Number of Newborn Affected
Birthmark	1 in 3
Down syndrome (mother age 29) (mother age 36)	1 in 1000 1 in 200
Heart defect	1 in 100
Polydactyly (extra fingers or toes)	50 in 100,000
Sickle-cell anemia	150 in 100,000 Afro-Americans
Spina bifida	1 in 1000

Structural birth defects such as those mentioned in the table are relatively rare—although they continue to be of concern to every potential mother and father. Parents, however, must also take into consideration other types of birth defects, such as the following:

- More than 7 percent of full-term newborns weigh less than 5.5 pounds (2500 grams), a low birth weight for gestational age that, according to the March of Dimes, puts the babies at 40 percent greater risk of dying during their first month of life than heavier babies.

- According to the Association for Retarded Citizens, about one out of every ten Americans has a family member with mental retardation. Approximately 2.6 million children have a mental disorder, and more than 100,000 babies are born with this type of defect each year. The known major causes of retardation are genetic conditions inherited from parents, disorders of genes caused by diseases or over-exposure to X rays, drugs, or chemicals during pregnancy, chromosomal abnormalities such as Down syndrome, or fragile X syndrome (an inherited break or weakness on a section of the X chromosome), and maternal alcoholism.

- According to the U.S. Department of Education, about 11 percent of all American schoolchildren are learning disabled and need special education.

These statistics highlight the fact that structural defects account for only a fraction of the total number of birth defects.

WHO'S AT RISK

Although birth defects appear in every population group in North America, the frequency and type of physical defects differ amongst races, ethnic groups, and socioeconomic groups. According to the CDC, Native Americans have the highest incidence of infant death within the first year of life due to major birth defects per 1000 total births (22.0), followed by whites (19.0), Afro-Americans (18.0), Asians (15.8), and Hispanics (14.4). These figures pertain only to structural defects.

Whether birth defects are structural or behavioral, however, figuring out who is at risk is not easy. Thanks to the Collaborative Perinatal Project, which studied more than 50,000 pregnancies from 1958 to 1965, we have part of the answer. The project data indicate that men were more likely to father a child with a birth defect if they themselves had a defect. Women were more likely to give birth to babies with birth defects if they fell into any of the following categories:

- During pregnancy were exposed to radiation, maternal infections, chemicals, vitamin and mineral excesses or deficiencies, or drugs
- Lacked prenatal care—especially with less than five prenatal visits to a medical professional
- Were over age thirty
- Weighed too much or too little before pregnancy
- Gained less than 16.5 pounds during pregnancy
- Had a prior stillbirth or at least three prior premature births
- Had already given birth to a child with a major malformation
- Suffered from toxemia during pregnancy, including excessive protein in the urine, hypertension, and convulsions
- Had diabetes or certain other medical conditions before pregnancy—such as cardiovascular disorders, hyperthyroidism, endocrine diseases, urinary tract infections, blood coagulation disorders, or bacterial infections during the second or third trimester
- Received an abdominal X ray during pregnancy
- Gave birth to a baby who had a low birth weight—the lower the birth weight, the greater the risk of malformations

THE CAUSES OF BIRTH DEFECTS

The causes of birth defects can be divided into three major categories: genetic influences that you may not be able to control (such as hemophilia or Down syndrome); environmental factors that you clearly have the possibility of controlling (such as your own smoking, your alcohol consumption, or an infection that you could cure before conceiving); interrelated genetic and environmental factors (for example, an environmental hazard that could damage an egg or sperm and lead to a genetic abnormality in the fetus).

To understand how these factors influence birth, we must examine the role that genetics plays in creating birth defects.

GENETICS AND BIRTH DEFECTS

The instant one sperm pierces the outer layers of an egg, a biochemical change in the egg's surface makes the egg impermeable to all other sperm. At that same instant, the merging of sperm and egg creates the basic blue-

print for a new human being—a blueprint composed of biological substances called chromosomes. Since problems with chromosomes are the
basis for many genetic birth defects, let's take a closer look.

Each chromosome contains a chain of biochemical substances called
nucleic acids, including a sugar (deoxyribose), a phosphate (phosphoric
acid), and four bases (adenine, guanine, cytosine, and thymine). This
chain is called DNA (which stands for deoxyribonucleic acid).

The DNA chain is represented by the shape of a ladder. Most of the
time this ladder is twisted into a double helix (Figure 1).

The important aspect of DNA as it relates to birth defects is the biochemical alphabet created by the sequencing of adenine, guanine, cytosine, and thymine along the ladder. Just as varying letters form words that
can be used for countless meanings, varying combinations of these four
substances along the DNA ladder form distinct units of inheritance,
called genes.

It is the complete sequence of genes that we refer to as an individual's
unique genetic code. It is this code that creates the potential for every
characteristic that makes us who we are—our gender, height, body build
and eye color, our inborn talents and capabilities, part of our emotional
makeup, our minute-by-minute biochemical functioning, and even our
vulnerability to certain illnesses.

Every time a cell reproduces, these twisted ladders of DNA in the cell
nucleus straighten up and break in two. Each half is then used as a tem-
plate for a mirror-image version of itself. Thus, an identical genetic code is
repeated in every cell of the body.

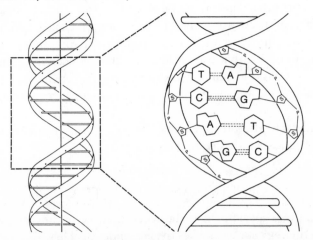

Figure 1. The double helix called DNA

In summary, the sequence of genes determines our genetic inheritance: Genes are located along twisted strands of DNA; DNA forms the structure called a chromosome; and chromosomes are found in the nucleus of body cells.

Sperm and egg cells each have twenty-three chromosomes. Since the human being results from a combination of one sperm and one egg, human cells contain forty-six chromosomes, or twenty-three pairs. One of each pair has been contributed by the father, and one by the mother.

Among the twenty-three pairs of chromosomes, one pair decides the sex of a child. Geneticists call the female gender chromosome the "X" chromosome, and the male gender chromosome the "Y" chromosome.

Each egg has one X chromosome. Of a man's sperm one-half have an X chromosome; the rest have a Y chromosome. The gender of a child depends on which sperm enters the egg. If sperm containing an X chromosome enters, the child will have two X chromosomes (one from the egg, one from the sperm) and will be female. If a sperm containing the Y chromosome enters, the child will have an X from the egg and the Y from the sperm, and be a male.

Chromosomal Mutations

Mutation simply means change, but most genetic mutations have a negative effect. Chromosomal mutations are one cause of birth defects. They are sometimes from unknown origin, sometimes the result of advanced age, and sometimes the result of environmental agents.

Occasionally, a child is born with an abnormal number of sex chromosomes. Some men, for instance, have a second female chromosome in addition to the usual X-and-Y pair that caused them to be male. This is called Klinefelter syndrome and can lead to physical and mental deficiencies. Some women have only one female-gender chromosome (called Turner syndrome) and may have learning disabilities and physical deformities.

Some people have too many or too few chromosomes among those chromosomes not related to gender. These abnormalities are due to improper cell division and cause various physical and mental effects. People with Down syndrome, for example, have an extra chromosome number 21.

Sometimes one part of a chromosome breaks off and attaches to another chromosome. People with this unusual chromosomal configuration often have no noticeable abnormalities. If they contribute that rearranged chromosome to a fetus, however, miscarriage may result, or their children may be born with apparent abnormalities.

These conditions are rare, as it is quite common for fetuses with severe chromosomal abnormalities to be miscarried. Fifteen to 20 percent of all pregnancies miscarry, and at least half of these miscarriages are caused by chromosomal abnormalities in the fetus.

Genetic Mutations

Chromosomes are composed of genes, and individual genes can also mutate, causing birth defects. Some genetic mutations, such as color blindness, are aggravating; some are fatal (for example, Tay-Sachs disease); and others are actually beneficial, such as tolerance for animal milk products. Genetic mutations may be expressed at birth, such as certain limb deformities, or they may reveal themselves over time only if conditions favor their expression, such as "fava-ism," which causes anemia if the person having this gene consumes fava beans. What genetic mutations have in common is their ability to be transmitted to the next generation when someone with the mutant gene has children.

Not all genetic mutations appear in the next generation. The appearance of inherited characteristics is determined by several factors. The primary one is chance. Your genetic inheritance reflects both your mother and your father (remember those twenty-three pairs of chromosomes)—a joint effect that is possible because each sperm and egg contain only one of every chromosome pair. It is a matter of chance which sperm and which egg unite to create the pairs that make you who you are.

The second-most important factor in genetic inheritance is the dominance of one gene over another.

Dominant traits.   Each of us inherits two separate sets of genes, one from each parent. These genes may indicate quite different, even contradictory, colors, textures, and sizes of body parts. We cannot be both red-headed and brunette or have long and short fingers at the same time, so nature has provided for an orderly choice of traits between our parents' two competing genetic codes. One of the most important determinants of heredity is the dominance of some genes over others.

Finger length is one good example. If you receive a gene for short fingers from your mother and long fingers from your father, you will have short fingers, because the genes for short fingers dominate the genes for long fingers. (Not long ago, biology students were taught that brown eyes dominated blue eyes, but now eye color is known to be more complicated than a case of simple dominance.)

Some abnormal conditions are inherited by simple dominance. When one parent passes on a dominant abnormal gene, even if the other parent contributes a gene for a normal corresponding body structure or function, the dominant gene will always express itself. For example, if a child receives a gene for achondroplasia (a common form of dwarfism) from one parent and a gene for a more common height from the other parent, he will have achondroplasia.

It does not matter how many children a couple has, or what their state of health, if one of the couple has a dominant gene, each child has a 50 percent chance of receiving that dominant gene.

Recessive traits.   With recessive traits, Mom and Dad must both contribute the same gene for a particular trait to be expressed in their child's body. For example, perhaps both your parents have short fingers, but you have long fingers. Because having long fingers is a recessive trait, your parents probably had no idea their genetic code harbored that trait until your long fingers appeared in the family. Your having long fingers means that on your mother's and your father's chromosomes the site dedicated to finger length must include one gene for long fingers in addition to the dominant one for short fingers. For you to exhibit long fingers, the gene contributed by your father and the one contributed by your mother must both be for long fingers.

Recessive genes for diseases are not usually pleasant surprises. For example, perhaps centuries ago, genetic mutations occurred in a few Jews in Eastern Europe. Not knowing they were passing on recessive genes with the potential for fatal diseases, such as Niemann-Pick, Tay-Sachs, and familial dysautonomia, carriers of the mutations continued to have children. Since Jews tended to marry Jews and tended to stay in the same village for generations, those mutant genes remained in the population's gene pool. Eventually, two people married who both carried a mutant recessive gene. In a similar process in Africa, the recessive mutated gene creating sickle-cell anemia remained unexpressed in the population's gene pool until two people who both carried the recessive gene for sickle-cell anemia married and had children. Sickle-cell anemia is only one of many diseases that are seen to be more prevalent in some population groups rather than others (see Table 2).

When two people carry the same mutant recessive gene and have a child, there is a 25 percent chance that the child will receive the mutant gene from both parents and express the symptom. There is also a 25 percent chance that the child will receive the dominant healthy gene from each parent (and therefore be not only completely healthy but also not be a carrier). There is a 50 percent chance that the child will receive one

Table 2. Genetic diseases prevalent among specific populations

Ethnic Group	Disease
Irish, Sikhs, and northern Chinese	neural tube defects
Afro-Americans	sickle-cell anemia
Jews	at least six different fatal diseases due to missing enzymes (proteins that speed up chemical reactions)
Mediterranean people (from Italy, Greece, N. Africa, Cyprus, Sardinia, Malta, Sicily, Rhodes, and parts of Turkey, India, and Southeast Asia)	thalassemia (a form of anemia) and G6PD deficiency (a missing enzyme)

mutant gene and one healthy gene, making that child a carrier but healthy. No matter how many children the couple have, and no matter whether the recessive gene in question is dangerous or benign, these percentages of risk repeat themselves for each child.

When a recessive genetic mutation appears only on the X chromosome, the physical or mental manifestation is apparent usually only in boys. Here's why: Since girls have two X chromosomes, a recessive gene on one will probably be mitigated by a normal matched gene on the other. Because boys have only one X chromosome, there is no other X to provide

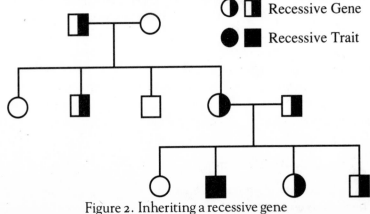

Figure 2. Inheriting a recessive gene

a normal matched gene to mitigate the mutant gene. This is why, more often than not, only boys have X-linked diseases, such as hemophilia, certain forms of muscular dystrophy, G6PD deficiency (a missing enzyme), and color blindness.

Geneticists estimate that all of us carry five to eight seriously disadvantageous recessive genes, but it is rare for two people with the same disadvantageous genes to have offspring together and to contribute the recessive gene for the same trait. In the case of Tay-Sachs, increased awareness of genetics and greater use of genetic counseling and blood testing have made the expression of this fatal genetic disease exceedingly rare among Jews.

Unfortunately, the major genetic disease among Afro-Americans, sickle-cell anemia, is still fairly widespread. With nearly one in ten Afro-Americans carrying the trait for sickle-cell anemia, nearly one in four hundred conceptions results in a child with the disease. A blood test reveals whether any one person is carrying the recessive gene for sickle-cell anemia.

The most common lethal recessive gene among whites is cystic fibrosis—a serious disease of the bowel and lungs. Although there is not yet routine screening for carriers of the gene, such screening may soon become available.

Other diseases based on single dominant or recessive genes include albinism (lack of the pigment melanin in skin, eyes, and hair), retinoblastoma (an eye tumor), familial hypercholesterolemia (high cholesterol), and PKU or phenylketonuria (absence of an enzyme needed to metabolize the amino acid phenylalanine).

Figure 2 indicates how an abnormal gene can be passed from one generation to another. In the first generation, one daughter and one son inherited the recessive abnormal gene (indicated by half black, half white symbols). That daughter unfortunately married a man with the same recessive abnormal gene. One of their daughters received the healthy, normal gene from both parents. Two children received the father's recessive abnormal gene and are, like their parents and maternal grandfather, carriers. One son received the abnormal gene from both parents, making him the only child in three generations who actually expresses the abnormal trait (for example, sickle cell anemia, albinism, or cystic fibrosis).

Diseases Based on Multiple Genes

There is also a class of inherited traits involving multiple genes. These traits express themselves only when certain external conditions occur.

Some examples of multiple-gene traits may surprise you; geneticists now include allergies, some cancers, asthma, hypertension, diabetes, and a large percentage of coronary-artery diseases in this category. The color of hair, eyes, and skin are hardly to be considered birth defects, but they, too, are now known to be the result of the influence of multiple genes.

Multiple-gene effects help explain why some smokers can smoke into their eighties, while others die in their forties. Our health is like a glass of water, filled partly by genetic inheritance and partly by environment. If you are graced with only one-quarter cup of the genes that contribute to disease, you can eat nonnutritious food or poison yourself with drugs and cigarettes for quite a while without noticeable ill effects. Eventually, however, you may affect that other three-quarter cupful of genetic inheritance, causing poor health. A different person may start with three-quarters of the inheritance loaded with genetic weaknesses; it thus takes less environmental input to elicit symptoms of ill health in that person.

Clues to multiple-gene traits abound in your own family history. If you add medical conditions to your family tree, do you find heart disease, diabetes, or cancer? This suggests an underlying genetic predisposition to certain illnesses that is unique to your family.

Some multiple-gene traits can be overridden by judicious therapy. For example, children with an abnormal need for a B vitamin called biotin are not able to recycle the vitamin the way normal people do because they lack an enzyme called biotinidase. Without biotin supplementation, these children sicken and die in early childhood. If they are given large doses of biotin on a regular basis, however, they do fine.

Genetic defects may affect the fetus in a wide variety of ways, depending on the particular defect and, in some cases, the interaction between the child and his environment. The effects range from miscarriage to no noticeable adverse symptoms whatsoever.

THE ENVIRONMENT AND BIRTH DEFECTS

Scientists are now examining the role that certain environmental agents, particularly chemicals and radiation, play in the development of birth defects. Unfortunately, the distinction between genetically caused and environmentally caused defects is fuzzy at times, since environmental dangers may induce a mutation in the sperm or the egg that later causes a genetic disorder in the child. This is new territory for scientists, and the connection between the two will be more clearly understood in coming years.

By looking at the process of conception in greater detail, we can see how environmental assaults on either parent—even before a child is conceived—may affect that child's well-being. We will begin with the woman, who holds within each of her ovaries 40,000 to 400,000 minuscule eggs—each in a sac called a follicle. These eggs formed while she, herself, was still within her mother's womb. A woman's own nine months as a fetus is, therefore, the first point at which exposure to environmental health hazards might permanently damage her eggs and thus affect her future children.

After a young woman reaches puberty, a hormone signals several follicles to grow and mature each month. One egg (sometimes more than one) matures beyond the others and, still in its follicle, moves to the surface of the ovary. About two weeks after the first day of a menstrual period, a second hormone causes the egg to burst through the walls of the follicle and ovary and to move into the nearby fallopian tube. The egg lives about forty-eight hours. If it is fertilized by a sperm in the fallopian tube during that time, it immediately begins to divide again and again, growing and developing for about three more days as it continues down the tube toward the uterus. About the time the next menstrual period is due, the egg implants itself on the wall of the uterus and builds an expandable fluid-filled cocoon called the amniotic sac in which it will float until birth. The embryo is attached to the placenta on one side of the amniotic sac by its umbilical cord, through which nutrients are absorbed and waste products are expelled. At any time during this process, chemical, nutritional, or other assaults on the egg's environment can interfere with normal cell division, implantation, and growth. During the next few weeks the heart, nervous system, eyes, ears, and limbs begin to appear. This is another critical time during which the developing fetus is vulnerable to environmental assault.

Let's now look at the man. When a man is a tiny embryo, his two sex glands—the testicles—develop inside his abdomen. By the time of birth the testicles usually have descended into the pouchlike scrotum outside his body. Like the woman, the man may be influenced by environmental agents even before his own birth. The testicles may have been influenced by exposure to radiation given to his mother, or by environmental toxins, such as chemicals to which his mother was exposed at work or at home.

When a man reaches puberty, the testicles begin producing the male hormone testosterone, which—along with hormones produced by the pituitary gland in the brain—initiates the production of sperm. From then on, sperm are continually manufactured inside the testicles. After their creation, sperm pass into a tightly coiled tube called the epididymis, where they continue their development for the next two to three weeks. It takes about ten weeks for sperm to reach full maturity.

Mature sperm are stored in the vas deferens, a long duct between each testicle and the urethra. If sperm are not ejaculated, they die, disintegrate, and are absorbed within the vas deferens. When a man ejaculates, the sperm move from the vas deferens into the urethra, where they are mixed with secretions from several nearby glands (including the prostate and seminal vesicles) that contain the proper nutrients to energize the sperm for their journey.

A man's reproductive health is as vulnerable to influence from the environment as is a woman's—especially since his contribution to conception is separated from the outside world by only a thin layer of skin. Fumes, chemicals, drugs, and radiation can alter the semen and sperm in unhealthy ways.

Although the environment can influence the reproductive systems of men and women while they are still fetuses, in this book I focus mainly on environmental agents, such as X rays, drugs, chemicals, nutritional deficiencies, and stress, that adversely affect adults who are trying to conceive. The degree of toxicity of environmental factors depends largely on the timing of exposure.

Timing of Exposure

During the first two weeks following fertilization, a developmental toxicant (any exposure, process, or event that alters the normal pattern of development) will generally either kill the new embryo or damage only a few cells, allowing the embryo to recover and develop without defects. From the fifteenth to the sixtieth day, however, the embryo is highly susceptible to malformations. Each organ and internal system has its own rhythm of development, and the exact date of exposure to any toxin has everything to do with which malformation will occur (see Table 3).

For example, a woman who contracts rubella (German measles) during her fourth week of pregnancy has a very high risk of giving birth to a child with congenital heart defects and cataracts. The same infection during her twenty-fourth week is very unlikely to create such problems.

Similarly, a potentially harmful drug taken during the early months of pregnancy may cause more all-encompassing damage than if the same drug were taken after the baby's organs, limbs, and major biochemical pathways have been formed. The brain, however, can be damaged throughout pregnancy, so a teratogen such as alcohol taken in excess at any time during pregnancy may cause behavioral or developmental problems.

Table 3. The effect of teratogens on the developing human

Time of exposure in weeks	Structure that may be altered
conception–2	none or death of embryo
end of 2–end of 6	heart
3–7	limbs
3–16	central nervous system
4–5	neural tube
4–8	eyes
4–9	ears
end of 6–9	palate
end of 6 to end of 9	genitalia
any time during pregnancy	brain
18 weeks prenatal to 8 years	teeth darkened by the antibiotic tetracycline

Age of the Parents

Age, which can be considered an environmental factor, appears to have an impact on the incidence of birth defects. For example, there is a higher incidence of gastrointestinal defects in children born to women younger than the age of twenty and a higher incidence of chromosomal defects, such as Down syndrome, in children of mothers over the age of thirty-five. Although the risk of giving birth to a baby with Down syndrome is greater with advancing maternal (and, some studies have indicated, paternal) age, women younger than age thirty-five are more fertile, have more babies, and consequently account for 80 percent of babies with Down syndrome in the population.

One simple explanation for the effect of a mother's age on the incidence of birth defects is that the older the egg, the more opportunity it has had to be exposed to noxious effects of chemicals, drugs, X rays, viruses, and other environmental agents.

Age, however, also pertains to the timing of fertilization. Some clinicians believe that the fertilization of an overripe egg can lead to a higher risk of malformations. An egg can become overripe by remaining in the ovary longer than usual before ovulation. This can occur at the beginning or end of a woman's fertile years; or after giving birth, having an abortion, having an overly long previous menstruation or a viral infection, or experiencing emotional stress.

An egg may also become overripe if intercourse takes place after ovulation and the egg has remained in the fallopian tubes a relatively long time before fertilization occurs. Therefore, according to this theory, the ideal timing of intercourse would be before you anticipate ovulation so sperm would already be in the fallopian tube when the egg arrives.

It is probably safe to say, however, that the majority of human beings alive and well today were conceived under less than optimum conditions. People have not always calculated their lovemaking to produce healthy babies, and they have exposed themselves to all manner of substances at every stage of pregnancy. This does not mean you ought to ignore environmental hazards and the other issues raised throughout this book, but you must recognize that many dangers have thresholds of toxicity. Exposure to levels below that threshold is thought to carry no additional risk. You can take the precautions that seem reasonable within the context of your daily life, while recognizing that birth defects may result from an interrelationship of genetic and environment factors, some of which you can control, and some you cannot.

PRENATAL TESTING FOR BIRTH DEFECTS

There are five commonly used tests, performed at various stages of pregnancy, to alert couples to possible reasons for concern or to assure them that their developing infant does not have specific defects. The tests are genetic counseling, blood tests, ultrasound, amniocentesis, and chorionic villus sampling.

Testing is especially useful in certain cases: for example, if you or someone in your family has already given birth to a child with a genetic defect, or if you are over age thirty-five, have diabetes, or know you were exposed to a toxic substance at a high dose or for a long period of time. Tests are also used when your doctor has reason to be concerned about a certain condition, such as abnormal fetal size or heart sounds.

Genetic Counseling

The advantage of genetic counseling is that it can be done before you become pregnant. By studying the medical conditions that appear on your family tree, a genetic counselor can help gauge the statistical likelihood of inherited diseases in your children. As a result, you can conceive with more confidence, or you may conclude you had best not conceive but should pursue alternative means of parenting, such as donor insemination or adoption. Or, you may decide to conceive and obtain one or more of the tests described in this book. Your physician, local March of Dimes office, or a major medical center can help you obtain genetic counseling.

Blood Tests

There are several blood tests available today that can help detect birth defects. A simple blood test, for example, can reveal a number of recessive genetic traits, including Tay-Sachs and sickle-cell anemia.

Another blood test can measure Maternal Serum Alpha-fetoprotein (MSAFP). Alpha-fetoprotein (AFP), a protein produced by the fetus, can be measured in the serum (watery part) of a mother's blood between her fifteenth and twentieth week of pregnancy. Higher than normal levels of AFP in the serum may indicate spina bifida, anencephaly, certain kidney or gastrointestinal problems, threatened or current miscarriage, or the presence of more than one fetus.

MSAFP testing is especially important in the case of neural tube defect (a collective name for anencephaly and spina bifida), since about 95 percent of infants born with NTD are born into families with no previous history of the problem. Pregnant women younger than thirty-five, who do not routinely undergo amniocentesis, can use MSAFP testing to learn if they are at increased risk for this condition.

In some cases, levels of maternal serum alpha-fetoprotein may seem abnormally high or low because of a mistake in calculating the due date. In addition, about 50 out of every 1000 women having the test will be told there may be a problem when they are carrying a normal child; approximately 100 out of every 1000 carrying a child with neural tube defect will be told the test is normal. If your results are abnormally high, you will probably be advised to retake the test or to have an ultrasound or amniocentesis to confirm the diagnosis.

One fairly uncommon test looks promising for diagnosing Down syndrome, especially for women younger than thirty-five. The test measures three different biological substances in the mother's blood during the second trimester of pregnancy: the level of hCG (human chorionic gonadotropin), MSAFP, and unconjugated estriol (a form of the female hormone estrogen). High levels of hCG coupled with low levels of estriol indicate a greater risk that the woman may be carrying a child with Down syndrome. Combining this figure with information obtained by an MSAFP measurement gives a more sensitive appraisal of the situation than is possible with the MSAFP test alone.

Ultrasound

Ultrasound is a relatively safe, entirely painless method of diagnosis that uses high-frequency sound waves.

A technician coats your belly with a gel to help conduct sound waves, then moves the ultrasound scanner gently against the skin. Inside the scanner is a crystal that changes electrical current into sound waves. The waves pass through the belly and reflect echoes from the structures they encounter, which are transformed into a black-and-white moving picture on a television monitor. You are awake and watching while this is occurring. The technician can point out your baby's head and backbone. Inspecting the baby's body in this way allows the physician to evaluate the baby's size and position and to learn whether you are carrying twins.

Structural birth defects such as anencephaly, some cases of spina bifida, and sometimes even heart abnormalities may be diagnosed using ultrasound, as can a number of other serious conditions. If there is suspicion of a heart defect, your physician will probably order an echocardiogram, a special form of ultrasound that readily diagnoses heart malfunctions and defects.

Ultrasound takes from fifteen minutes to an hour and may be performed at any stage of pregnancy. There may be some discomfort only if you are asked to maintain a full bladder during the procedure. If you ask, the technician can provide you with your first photo of your child, though to your untrained eyes the fetus will probably resemble, as one poetic observer says, a weather forecast for cloudy skies.

Around 40 to 60 percent of pregnant American women receive ultrasound. Although some studies have suggested that changes in tissues may take place at the cellular level, no effect has been documented. In fact, ultrasound has been used for twenty-five years in the United States without clear evidence of long-term harm to the mother or baby. Nevertheless, ultrasound is to be used only when medically necessary.

Amniocentesis

Ultrasound is a useful tool in its own right, but it is also an invaluable aid in performing amniocentesis. Amniocentesis has been used in the United States since the 1970s and is a relatively safe, reliable method of discovering whether a fetus has any of dozens of possible abnormalities, including Tay-Sachs disease, spina bifida, anencephaly, Down syndrome, and hemophilia. When done late in pregnancy, it can also reveal such problems as inadequate development of the lungs.

Amniocentesis is the removal, by syringe, of about four teaspoons or more of amniotic fluid (the watery substance in which the baby floats). The test is usually performed when you are around fifteen weeks pregnant and begins with an ultrasound, which pinpoints the location of the placenta and of the fetus. Guided by the ultrasound picture, the doctor inserts a needle through the abdomen and uterine wall and into the amniotic sac. Sometimes local anesthesia is used, but even without it the procedure is not especially uncomfortable.

The sampling procedure is over quite quickly. The hardest part is waiting for the results. It takes two weeks or longer for technicians to analyze the sample. This test is done during the second trimester, so if test results lead you to end your pregnancy, that process is a bit more involved than it would be during the first twelve weeks.

Amniocentesis results in a slightly increased risk of miscarriage, leakage of fluid, infection, or bleeding, but these are rare—as are any effects on the fetus. Amniocentesis is usually offered to women over the age of thirty-four or to those at higher than normal risk of miscarrying or having a baby with a chromosomal or congenital abnormality.

Chorionic Villus Sampling (CVS)

Introduced in the United States in 1983, Chorionic Villus Sampling (CVS) has become firmly established as a relatively accurate and safe means of genetic screening. Its biggest attraction is how early it can be performed—from weeks nine to twelve—and how quickly results can be returned (within hours or up to two weeks).

With CVS, a physician usually directs a tube with a syringe attached into the uterus through the vagina and draws up some tiny waving projections called villi from the surface of the amniotic sac, called the chorion. Sometimes, the villi are extracted with a hollow needle inserted through the abdominal wall. In most cases, these villi contain the same genetic code as does the fetus, allowing technicians to analyze them for genetic diseases and chromosomal abnormalities.

Since CVS is performed too early in a pregnancy to include MSAFP testing, it will not reveal a neural tube defect or other structural defects. For a forty-year-old mother, however, the risk of a chromosome abnormality is ten to twenty-five times greater than is her risk of having a child with neural tube defect, so a CVS procedure can be an important source of information.

Although in the vast majority of cases CVS is perfectly safe, researchers have found a statistically measurable increased risk of limb abnormalities, including missing or shortened fingers, among mothers who had CVS compared to the general population. Thus, as with all prenatal tests, the decision to use CVS ought to be made after careful discussion with your obstetrician about its risk and accuracy in your case.

The information you receive from prenatal testing gives you time to consider your options and, as a couple, to commit yourselves to whatever choices you make, including whether to begin a pregnancy and, once a pregnancy is established, whether to continue it.

Before you consent to any prenatal testing, ask questions and know the reason for your particular test, the possible risks to you or your fetus, and whether the doctor or you would handle the pregnancy differently if a particular test was positive. Doctors may need your test results to decide how best to manage the pregnancy and birth.

For many women, waiting for results can be a time of great upset and fear. It can also be an opportunity to get in touch with the fetus and your partner in greater depth than ever before. Tests force you both to confront what you might have put off as too scary or uncomfortable, but often by facing them you can move into a new level of partnership.

The remaining chapters of this book present actions that you can take to ensure the healthiest conditions for conception, pregnancy, birth, and beyond.

PART ONE

Before Pregnancy

Preconception Care

E ven before sperm meets egg, you can take steps that help ensure the health of your baby. A growing enthusiasm for prevention-oriented medical care has produced a new movement among health professionals called preconception care. It requires, for example, that the mother-to-be make a conscious decision to eat more nutritiously, to reduce or eliminate her use of medications several months before becoming pregnant, and to plan the pregnancy instead of being pleasantly surprised.

The premier example of successful preconception care is reported by a nonprofit British organization named Foresight, The Association for the Promotion of Preconceptual Care. In 1978, Foresight created a program that is now followed by about forty physicians throughout Great Britain. Collectively, Foresight patients have a low (.37 percent) rate of birth defects, compared to 6 to 7 percent, which is the national average in England and America. They also have one-fourth the rate of miscarriage and prematurity, and they reported no infant deaths during the past ten years.

Foresight's basic tenets derive from the work of Arthur and Margaret Wynn, who reviewed the reproductive history of people who had experienced famine, been exposed to radiation, or used medicinal drugs excessively. They concluded that a minimum of four months prior to conception is needed for the body to recover from specific exposure to mutagenic substances or long-term nutritional deficiencies. In addition, the Foresight program draws heavily upon other pioneering research that reveals the critical role of parental nutrition in compensating for environmentally induced deficiencies and other clinical conditions.

During the four to six months of preconception work, Foresight's participants undergo the following:

• an evaluation of both partners' nutritional habits, with appropriate revision of their diet to add missing nutrients

- hair analysis to detect heavy-metal poisoning or trace-mineral deficiencies
- elimination of heavy-metal poisoning or trace-metal deficiencies through diet and supplementation
- diagnosis and treatment of allergies
- clearing genitourinary infections and controlling other infections, such as cytomegalovirus, Candida albicans, rubella, or toxoplasmosis in both men and women
- weaning off pharmaceuticals, alcohol, cigarettes, and caffeine
- filtration of all drinking water
- assistance in reducing emotional stress
- for the male partner, testing sperm number and sperm quality and treating unhealthy levels of abnormal sperm with zinc, manganese, vitamin E, vitamin B-12, a general B complex, potassium, plus all the previously mentioned therapeutics
- use of natural family-planning methods, including such barrier devices as a condom, diaphragm, or cervical cap during the fertile phase each month until all the above cleansing programs are completed

From Encino, California, to Quakerstown, Pennsylvania, American physicians, too, are beginning to appreciate preventive obstetrics. At the University of North Carolina at Chapel Hill's Department of Maternal-Fetal Medicine, American preconception pioneers Dr. Robert Cefalo and nurse-practitioner Merry-K. Moos have developed a form called the Preconceptional Health Appraisal to help women who are not yet pregnant to figure out what in their lifestyles may need revision. Use of the appraisal has spread to private medical clinics and health departments across the country.

Preconception care is a cost-effective and unsuccessful way to prevent some problems, but it is up to you to initiate changes in your lifestyle that will make the difference in your pregnancy and birth.

· W H A T   T O   D O ·

☑ Enlist the help of your physician to create a preconception plan for you and your mate. You will need to look at every aspect of your daily life, including your diet; use of medications; consumption of coffee, soda, alcohol, and cigarettes; water quality; and any health problems you may need to correct before pregnancy, such as urogenital infections or uncontrolled diabetes. If you need professional help to stop smoking or consuming alcohol, get it. And, do not leave out the father-to-be. Research has indicated that a father's drinking and smoking during the months just prior to conception can affect the health of his child.

You will also want to get a blood test to check not only your immunity to various infectious diseases, such as rubella, but also the level of lead in your blood. Lead, a common pollutant in some house paints and old plumbing, diminishes the intelligence of children who are exposed to it in the womb. You may also wish to have your blood tested for pesticide residues. These diagnostic steps are equally important for both the mother- and the father-to-be.

✔ If you are not sure what aspects of your life may need changing, you may find the computer-scored questionnaire called Before Pregnancy Health Inventory quite useful. This patient-education tool is adapted from the original questionnaire designed at the University of North Carolina at Chapel Hill. After completing the Inventory, you will receive a custom-designed twenty- to thirty-page guide that details the changes you ought to make. A short summary of the guide will be sent to your physician to help you create a medically supervised preconception plan. Order the questionnaire from Before Pregnancy Health Inventory, Perinatal Health, Inc., 7777 Greenback Lane, Apt. 205, Citrus Heights, Calif. 95610, 916-725-4035. Cost: $44 to you directly; $36 through a physician.

✔ Stop taking birth-control pills (if you are using this method of contraception) at least three months before you desire to conceive. Birth-control pills can deplete the body of folic acid, certain B vitamins, vitamin C, vitamin E, manganese, and zinc. Use alternative birth-control methods during these three months.

✔ Start taking prenatal vitamin supplements. According to the U.S. Department of Agriculture, many American women eat nutritionally inadequate diets and need extra help in preparing their bodies for pregnancy.

In some women, supplements seem to prevent the spinal malformation called neural tube defect. According to a study conducted by the Centers for Disease Control in 1988, prenatal multivitamins containing folic acid have the greatest impact when taken at the time of conception and through the early weeks of pregnancy.

- ☑ If you have uncontrolled diabetes, you are at risk of having a child with a birth defect, but if you can enter pregnancy with blood sugar already under control, the risk drops to that of a woman who does not have diabetes.

- ☑ If you have any diagnostic X rays, be sure your ovaries (or testes, for men) are shielded from direct beams with leaded covers and that when possible the technician reduces the radiation field size to protect your reproductive organs from the inevitable scattering of radiation.

- ☑ The Foresight recommendations listed in this chapter offer a basic outline. For more specific advice and a copy of *For Tomorrow's Children* (the Foresight program's instructional guide, edited for an American audience) write to Harold Buttram, M.D., Preconception Care, Inc., P.O. Box 357, Blooming Glen, Penn. 18911, 215-536-1890.

- ☑ You can find out more about Foresight publications by sending a self-addressed envelope to Foresight, The Old Vicarage, Church Lane, Witley, Surrey, GU8 5PN, England.

Pre-existing Medical Conditions

I f you know you have a serious pre-existing medical condition, it is especially important to discuss your goal of pregnancy with a physician and to take whatever steps are necessary to minimize the effects of both the disease itself and any medication you take for it before becoming pregnant. In this chapter we will examine three conditions that are of special concern for the parent-to-be: AIDS, diabetes, and epilepsy.

AIDS

In 1979, doctors in New York and Los Angeles noticed unusual illnesses in a small number of homosexuals in those cities. In 1981, the Centers for Disease Control began recording cases of the condition that was later to be called Acquired Immune Deficiency Syndrome. It is not actually a disease but a group of problems suspected to be the result of infection by human immunodeficiency virus (HIV). The virus debilitates a person's immune system, making the body more susceptible to other infections. Many of these opportunistic infections normally would not be dangerous, but in the HIV-infected person they become major assaults on health.

HIV is usually acquired when semen, vaginal fluid, or blood from an infected person passes into the bloodstream of another person through oral, vaginal, or anal sex. Intravenous drug users are at high risk because the virus can also be spread through infected needles and syringes. Others at risk are those receiving multiple blood transfusions, or who received transfusions before 1988, when most blood banks began screening closely for HIV-positive blood.

More than 2600 children in the United States younger than age thirteen have developed AIDS as of 1991. Some were born prematurely, have hemophilia, or for some other reason received HIV-tainted blood during transfusions. The vast majority of children with AIDS were infected by their mothers during pregnancy or delivery. However, around 70 percent of newborns who initially test positive will actually, months later, test negative for HIV. The false positive is due to the time it takes for healthy newborns to clear maternal antibodies from their system.

· W H A T   T O   D O ·

☑ If you are planning to become pregnant and have been with other sexual partners during the past dozen years, you and your mate may want to talk to a doctor or an AIDS-test counselor about taking the test for HIV antibodies. This test checks the blood for evidence of past exposure to the virus associated with AIDS.

  The U.S. Public Health Service provides a free twenty-four-hour hotline to answer questions and to tell you the location of a confidential testing center near you: 800-342-AIDS; Hearing Impaired, 800-AIDS-TTY.

  If you are a woman who has developed pelvic inflammatory disease (PID), human papilloma virus (vaginal warts), or other signs of a sexually transmitted disease (STD), it may be an especially good idea for you to obtain HIV antibody testing (in addition to clearing up your STD) before pregnancy.

DIABETES

If you have diabetes, you, more than many women, are used to speedy feedback from your body when you do not eat what is right for you. Eating too much, too little, or the wrong food plays havoc with your blood sugar, and you have to correct the situation or suffer severe consequences. Self-care is vitally important, not only to you but also to your developing fetus. It can make the difference between serious problems and none at all.

You probably already know that having diabetes means that your pancreas does not produce adequate insulin or that your body cannot use the insulin that is produced as effectively as needed. Since insulin's job is to allow the glucose (sugar) in your bloodstream to enter body cells and be used for energy, inadequate insulin causes the blood sugar to build up until your kidneys cannot filter it as they normally do. Tests may reveal traces of glucose in your urine.

Excessive glucose in the blood and extracellular fluid causes frequent urination and severe thirst; lack of glucose in the cells causes weight loss and fatigue. Abnormal fat metabolism, cardiovascular disease, kidney disease, loss of vision, and reduced circulation and nerve sensitivity in the toes and fingers are some common complications resulting from diabetes.

If you have Type 2 (noninsulin-dependent) diabetes (formerly called adult-onset diabetes), your pancreas may produce some insulin but not enough to keep your blood sugar at a normal level, or your body may not use its insulin properly. Approximately 20 pregnancies in 1000 in the United States involve women who have Type 2 diabetes.

About 2 pregnancies in 1000 in the United States occur in women who have Type 1 (insulin-dependent) diabetes (formerly called juvenile diabetes). This type of diabetes must be carefully monitored to control the blood sugar. The developing baby makes extra demands on your body's energy supply. If insulin is not available to provide cells with the glucose they need, fat may be used instead of glucose; this condition produces acidic compounds called ketones. In excess, these acids can be toxic, leading to a serious condition called ketoacidosis. Not only might you go into a coma, but your baby may also be threatened with damage, even death. Careful control of blood-sugar levels can prevent this.

Women with Type 1 diabetes are also at risk of miscarriages, preeclampsia (a severe toxic condition during pregnancy), preterm labor, and stillbirths. Their babies, moreover, may be born with a calcium deficiency, liver dysfunction, hypoglycemia, or structural birth defects—particularly those affecting the heart, spinal column, brain, lungs, liver, kidneys, or gastrointestinal tract.

In the past, infants of women with diabetes often died if the pregnancy was allowed to continue past thirty-eight weeks, so cesarean section was commonly performed. Today, most women who maintain good blood-glucose control during pregnancy can experience a vaginal delivery.

Frequently, babies born to mothers with diabetes are larger than other babies and have more fragile health. Too much glucose in the baby's bloodstream may lead to respiratory distress. These newborns are commonly treated as carefully as if they were premature.

Self-care does not stop with delivery. Since diabetes tends to run in families, your pediatrician may want to keep close watch on your baby's blood sugar. Scientists now believe that both forms of diabetes develop in an individual who was born with a tendency toward the condition after a viral infection alters the normal immune response and causes the child's body to destroy its own insulin-producing cells. In some cases, this occurs before birth during a mother's infection with rubella (German measles); in other cases, it occurs during childhood.

The incidence of diabetes among the children of parents with insulin-dependent diabetes ranges from over 1 percent for children of mothers with the insulin-dependent form of the disease, to over 6 percent for children of fathers with the same condition. From 15 to 25 percent of the children of parents with noninsulin-dependent diabetes develop diabetes some time later in their lives.

· W H A T   T O   D O ·

☑ Before pregnancy, get your blood sugar under tight control. Preconception planning prevents a fluctuating blood sugar from damaging your child during the early weeks of organ formation, which usually occurs before you know you are pregnant. In a study by John L. Kitzmiller, M.D., women with diabetes who controlled their blood sugar from before pregnancy through delivery showed no greater level of birth defects or adverse pregnancy outcome than did women who do not have diabetes. Among those with diabetes who began self-care later in pregnancy, 11 percent delivered babies with defects, compared to 2 percent in the preconception-care group.

☑ If you have unprotected intercourse, assume you are pregnant until proven wrong and be extra cautious in controlling your blood sugar.

☑ Choose an obstetrician who specializes in high-risk pregnancies. Coordinate your preconception care with your endocrinologist. Consult them before consuming any medication, even nonprescription medication.

✓ Since women with diabetes are at special risk of genitourinary tract infections, obtain routine screening for these conditions and do not get pregnant until you are free of infection.

✓ Stop taking oral hypoglycemic drugs once you have become pregnant, as they have been associated with severe hypoglycemia in newborns and are suspected of causing birth defects. If control of blood sugar by diet alone is not possible, you will most likely begin insulin therapy at this time.

✓ If your blood sugars are low (hypoglycemia), avoid situations that might be dangerous, such as driving alone, until your tests prove that your blood glucose is stable. It is common for pregnant women with insulin-dependent diabetes to have hypoglycemia during the first trimester, when the baby's need for your glucose contributes to other factors that may cause unexpected and sudden decreases in your blood sugar. Unfortunately, you may not be aware that you have slipped into hypoglycemia. That is why it is important to test your blood sugar frequently.

✓ Your baby's health depends to a great extent on your maintaining your blood sugar between 60 and 105 mg/dL before meals, between 100 and 160 mg/dL an hour after meals, and between 80 and 120 mg/dL two hours after meals. To do this, monitor yourself four to six times a day, using capillary–blood-glucose measurement strips or glucose meters. An automatic pricking device will make reliable testing easy, quick, and relatively comfortable. If your blood glucose measures outside these ranges, contact your physician.

✓ Test your urine for ketones before breakfast each morning and at other times during the day to decide which carbohydrates to consume.

✓ Contact your physician immediately if you notice any of the following signs of trouble: painful urination or any other indication of urogenital infection; unrelieved vomiting; severe headache; any change in vision; sudden swelling of face or fingers; any discharge from the vagina; severe abdominal pain; lack of fetal movement; or sudden drop in normal amount of fetal movement.

☑ Call the American Diabetes Association (800-232-3472) for a referral to an accredited diabetes-education program near you.

☑ For additional advice, read Thomas Brewer, M.D., and Gail Sforza Brewer's *Brewer Medical Diet for Normal and High-Risk Pregnancy* (Simon & Schuster 1983) and June Biermann, Barbara Toohey, and Dr. Lois Jovanovic's *The Diabetic Woman* (Tarcher 1987).

EPILEPSY

Epilepsy involves temporary alterations of brain function; this might include total loss of consciousness and spasmed muscles (grand mal seizures) or simply momentary losses of consciousness (petit mal seizures). The problem can result from many different diseases or injuries, including birth trauma, head injury, stroke, brain infections, a metabolic imbalance, or severe drug intoxication.

Seizures may be more frequent during pregnancy due to normal biochemical changes. They are dangerous for the fetus, as loss of oxygen during the seizure can lead to placental separation and even fetal death. Unfortunately, commonly prescribed anticonvulsant medications can cause birth defects. In studies, phenytoin—Dilantin®—caused birth defects in about one in ten fetuses exposed to it, while trimethadione—Tridione®—caused birth defects in as many as six out of ten exposed fetuses. Perhaps because of oxygen deprivation during seizures, women with epilepsy who do not take medication have a higher rate of birth defects than the general population but only one-third the risk of women on anticonvulsants. Men on anticonvulsants also have a higher risk of producing a baby with birth defects.

As serious as these statistics seem, more than 90 percent of women taking anticonvulsant medications give birth to healthy infants.

· W H A T   T O   D O ·

☑ Tell your gynecologist about any history of seizures, no matter how long ago they occurred. You may need to be evaluated by a specialist before you conceive; sometimes pregnancy will bring on a seizure in women who have not had any for many years.

- ☑ If you or your partner are currently on anticonvulsant medication, you are in the best position to prevent drug effects before conceiving. Alert your neurologist to your intentions. The neurologist will change your medication to the least teratogenic drug possible. New research indicates that taking only one anticonvulsant drug leads to fewer incidences of birth defects than multiple drug therapy. If you have not had a seizure in several years, your physician may gradually eliminate all your medication during pregnancy.

- ☑ For further information, contact the Epilepsy Foundation of America, 800-EFA-1000 or 301-459-3700, or the National Epilepsy Library, 4351 Garden City Drive, Landover, Md. 20785, 800-EFA-4050.

Occupational Hazards
for Women

M ore than half of all women ages eighteen to sixty-five are now working outside the home. If you are one of them, you are more likely to
work more during pregnancy and to stay on the job later into pregnancy
than did your mother and grandmother. Your salary is probably needed
to help pay the family's bills, and you are grateful to have a job. Toxicants
at your workplace, however, may interfere with conception, cause physical
or mental problems in your child, and pollute your milk after delivery.

A study conducted by the University of Oslo, Norway, compared birth
defects with the occupation of the mother and concluded that about 9 percent of birth defects are due to contaminants found in the workplace.
Studies conducted in the United States found that the most common
means of exposure to toxicants include inhaling vapors, absorbing toxicants through the skin, and swallowing toxicants that have contaminated
hands, food, drink, or cigarettes. Workers can also bring home toxic dust
on tools, skin, and clothing—thereby contaminating the whole family.

Most at risk for miscarriages, birth defects, or other undesired pregnancy outcomes are women who work in agricultural and chemical indus-
tries, on farms, at dry cleaning establishments, in food-and-drink indus-
tries, at glass- and pottery-manufacturing plants, as hairdressers, hospital
workers, jute and rope manufacturers, painters, printers, electronics manufacturing workers, textile workers, welders, and woodworkers.

What might these women be exposed to that is so dangerous? California was one of the first states to create a list of hazardous chemicals—
thanks to the Safe Drinking Water and Toxic Enforcement Act of 1986. I
have used its list as an example of the chemicals and drugs known to cause
reproductive harm to women and fetuses (see Table 4). (Those affecting

Table 4. Chemicals known to the State of California to cause reproductive harm, as of January 1, 1992 (excluding pharmaceuticals)

Developmental toxicity

Acetohydroxamic acid

Benzphetamine hydrochloride

Bischloroethyl nitrosourea (BCNU) (Carmustine)

Bromoxynil

1,4-Butanedio dimethylsulfonate (Busulfan)

Carbon disulfide

Carbon monoxide

Chenodiol

Chlorcyclizine hydrochloride

Chlordecone (Kepone)

1-(2-Chloroethyl)-3-cyclohexyl-1-nitrosourea (CCNU) (Lomustine)

Cynazine

Cycloheximide

Cyhexatin

Dinocap

Dinoseb

Ethyl alcohol in alcoholic beverages

Ethylene glycol monoethyl ether

Ethylene glycol monomethyl ether

Hexachlorobenzene

Iodine

Lead

Mercury, mercury compounds, and methyl mercury

Methacycline hydrochloride

Mitroxantrone hydrochloride

Nicotine

Pipobroman

Polychlorinated biphenyls

Procarbazine hydrochloride

2, 3, 7, 8-Tetrachlorodibenzo-para-dioxin (TCDD)

Tobacco smoke (primary)

Toluene

Female reproductive toxicity

Carbon disulfide

Ethylene oxide

Lead

Tobacco smoke (primary)

Source: State of California Safe Drinking Water and Toxic Enforcement Act of 1986

men are discussed in "The Father's Role.") Developmental toxicity means the substance can alter normal development of either a fetus or a child. Reproductive toxicity means the substance can affect the structure and function of the reproductive system (including damage to a woman's eggs, which might lead to defective embryos and miscarriage).

In some cases, childhood cancer originates in maternal or paternal exposure to a toxicant even before pregnancy began. So, even if you are not yet pregnant, you must take steps to reduce or eliminate exposure to the toxicants that are known to affect the reproductive system.

· W H A T   T O   D O ·

☑ If you suspect that you are exposed to toxic substances, you will need to identify the substance and the degree of exposure. Then you must determine if any evidence exists that links the substances in question with adverse reproductive effects. Thanks to a federal Hazards Communication Standard and state right-to-know laws, upon request you or your health provider must be supplied material-safety data sheets that will tell you the potential side effects of substances to which you are exposed on the job. Ask for additional information from your company's medical department, your union, or the manufacturer of the substance.

You can also ask a library connected with a local hospital, medical school, or county medical society to do a computerized search of the medical literature for you—once you know what substances you want to research. At the library, you may find the *Catalog of Teratogenic Agents* (1989), by Thomas H. Shepard, M.D., useful. If you own a personal computer, you can use Rachel (Remote Access Chemical Hazards Electronic Library), which is a free database containing information about hazardous materials. Rachel is provided to the public by the Environmental Research Foundation, P.O. Box 73700, Washington, D.C. 20056-3700, 202-328-1119.

☑ Find out if the hazards in your workplace include known carcinogenic chemicals, even if their reproductive effects have not yet been proven. Avoid exposure to these before and during pregnancy. A great deal of evidence exists linking carcinogens (which cause cancer) and mutagens (which cause mutations, or changes in genes that might lead to birth defects).

☑ Protect yourself. When alerted by your obstetrician or another medical authority, an employer may be willing to change the workplace to protect your health (such as providing alternative, less-toxic materials, better isolation of dangerous substances, improved ventilation, and supplies—such as an apron and gloves or a respirator that can help you stay clear of exposure) or to transfer you to a safer work environment with equal wages and benefits. So, talk to your personal physician about your concerns.

☑ Inform yourself. Two sources of information on environmental and occupational health issues are:

Resource Center, Public Education and Risk Communication Division, Environmental and Occupational Health Sciences Institute, Brookwood II, 45 Knightsbridge Road, Piscataway, N.J. 08854, 201-463-5353. (The center offers fact sheets, videos, resource guides, and more.)

National Safe Workplace Institute, 122 South Michigan Avenue, Apt. 1450, Chicago, Ill. 60603, 312-939-0690. (The institute publishes studies of issues that pertain to health and safety in the workplace.)

THE WOMAN WORKING AT HOME

You cannot forget that you work in the home, even if you do not work for a paycheck. Housework puts you in contact with toxic chemicals, such as petroleum distillates, benzene, naphtha, chlorinated hydrocarbons, and ammonia. These can be hazardous to you and your developing baby before and during pregnancy. In the mid-1980s, a report by the Consumer Product Safety Commission identified 150 chemicals—pollutants linked with cancer, allergies, psychological abnormalities, and birth defects—regularly found in homes. The report warns that indoor pollution is worsening.

· W H A T   T O   D O ·

☑ Take a look beneath your kitchen sink. It is probably one of the most dangerous areas in your house. How many labels carry the warning *Poison: May be fatal or cause permanent damage if swallowed?* Throw them all away.

☑ Simplify your housecleaning by using natural supplies, such as a mixture of vinegar, lemon, and water; lots of baking soda; chlorine-free Bon Ami cleaning powder; borax; and steel wool. That is all you need to keep a home spotless. For excellent advice on safe housekeeping, read:

   Nontoxic, Natural, & Earthwise (Tarcher 1991), by Debra Lynn Dadd.

   Clean & Green: 485 Ways to Clean, Polish, Disinfect, Deodorize, Launder, Remove Stains—Even Wax Your Car Without Harming Yourself or the Environment (Ceres Press 1990), by Annie Berthold-Bond. You may order this book for $8.95, plus $2 for shipping, from Ceres Press, P.O. Box 87, Dept. BD, Woodstock, N.Y. 12498, 914-679-5573.

The Father's Role

M en can contribute to an adverse pregnancy in three important ways. First, fathers are part of the expectant mother's emotional environment, which can affect birth weight and the risk of prematurity. Second, men can inadvertently contaminate mothers-to-be, newborns, and growing children by bringing home toxic dust from the workplace on their clothes and tools. Third, the man's crucial contribution to the pregnancy is his production of healthy sperm, but sperm are susceptible to the effect of environmental agents, such as drugs, chemicals, and radiation. It is this third factor that we will explore in this chapter.

AGE AND INHERITANCE

Most people have heard that pregnant women over the age of forty are a high-risk group. Paternal age, however, is known to contribute to the development of at least a dozen types of genetic defects in children. Some of the abnormal conditions that result from genetic changes in the sperm of fathers who are forty years of age or older include Marfan syndrome (abnormally long and flexible fingers and limbs and anomalies of the eyes and the heart), Lesch-Nyhan syndrome (physical and mental retardation with spastic movements), and achondroplasia (a common form of dwarfism).

According to researcher Jan M. Friedman, M.D., Ph.D., at the University of British Columbia in Vancouver, about one-third of all babies with diseases due to new single-gene mutations (those not inherited from previous generations) are fathered by men forty years of age or older.

Scientists have found that from 5 to 20 percent of the cases of Down syndrome, a chromosomal aberration, result from defective sperm, but not every study on the subject has found a clear connection between paternal age and increased risk of Down syndrome. In general, older men have children with older women, so it has been difficult for researchers to single out the father's age as the causal factor producing this condition.

ENVIRONMENTAL INFLUENCES ON SPERM

Our understanding of the influence of the environment on the male re-productive system began more than two hundred years ago, with the observed increase in testicular cancer among chimney sweeps. We now know that toxic substances can also reduce the overall number of sperm, increase the number of abnormal sperm, decrease sperm motility (the ability of sperm to move with whiplike motions), or reduce the quantity of semen that nourishes the sperm.

Mother Nature does her best to protect the male reproductive system, but her efforts are not perfect. Sperm are produced in the seminiferous tubules, which are long, convoluted, and composed of cells so tightly squeezed together that they form an effective barrier to many chemical and drug hazards. Some substances, however, can penetrate the tubules. For example, according to Russell Davis, Ph.D., at the University of California, Davis, Division of Reproductive Biology and Medicine, when pilots of crop duster planes provide a sperm sample, the sample literally reeks of pesticides. The abnormalities potentially produced may be minor or severe, depending on whether individual genes or parts of whole chromosomes are damaged, and how much damage is done, and may involve spontaneous abortion, birth defects, abnormal fetal growth, neonatal death, developmental problems and learning disabilities, and childhood cancer.

In addition, toxicants can reduce the number of sperm produced. The average American male today has between 50 and 70 million sperm per milliliter of semen. A sperm count below 20 million per milliliter is considered abnormally low. In 1949 two studies found the average sperm count of American men was over 140 million sperm per milliliter of semen. From 1969 to 1979 only one study in sixteen found an average sperm count over 98 million. Nevertheless, researchers do not believe that American men's sperm count has dramatically decreased. Instead, they relate the above differences to changes in laboratory techniques during the last fifty years and on a change in the population of males studied, from college students to an older population of men visiting infertility clinics.

Besides drugs and chemicals, other factors can damage sperm production, including severe emotional distress, infections, and excessive heating of the body (hyperthermia). One study found it took three months for sperm production to return to prehyperthermia levels—so trying to get your wife pregnant in a hot tub is probably not a good idea.

It is important to realize, however, that the quality of sperm plays a greater role than the number in congenital malformations and functional problems, cautions Cappy Rothman, M.D., cofounder and director of The

California Cryobank (a major sperm bank in California). In extreme cases the quantity of sperm becomes important. Men with less than 20 million sperm per milliliter of semen commonly have significantly more chromosomal aberrations than do men with higher sperm counts.

The following is a review of the three major environmental influences on male reproductive health: drugs, chemicals, and radiation.

Drugs

Drugs are a potent environmental toxicant affecting semen. Since the woman's body absorbs the semen, reports in the medical literature have cited women receiving doses of pharmaceuticals that are dangerous to a fetus through their partners' semen. For example, children have been born deformed after their fathers, not their mothers, took drugs such as thalidomide or an anticonvulsant.

Here's a summary of the effect specific drugs can have on the man's reproductive health:

Alcohol.   Most women know that drinking during pregnancy can harm the fetus. New studies suggest that even drinking before conception—by fathers and mothers—may be a bad idea. Drs. Ruth Little and Charles Sing found that when a father averaged two or more drinks a day or at least five drinks on one occasion in the month prior to conception, a baby's birth weight was nearly 5 ounces less than that of babies of nondrinking fathers.

Some research also suggests that sons are especially susceptible to damage from alcohol, whether the offending parent is the father or the mother. Sons of alcoholics suffer hormonal imbalances and more trouble with schoolwork than do either their sisters or the sons of nonalcoholics.

Cigarettes.   A father's smoking habits affect not only his testosterone and sperm motility but also the fetus, according to German studies. Researchers noted that specific facial malformations in children were related to the quantity of smoking done by the father before and during pregnancy. Other studies have reported more babies with a low birth weight and increased death and congenital defects among babies of fathers who smoked cigarettes. Increased risk of brain cancer and leukemia have also been reported for children of fathers who smoke.

Marijuana.   Frequent use of marijuana may decrease fertility, as it can lower sperm motility and sperm count, increase sperm abnormalities and, after chronic use, may cause impotence. There is little proof that the drug causes birth defects. One estimate suggests that about one-fourth of the American population has at some time smoked marijuana. Its major active ingredient, tetrahydrocannabinol (THC), tends to accumulate in fat cells and is only slowly eliminated from the body.

Prescription drugs.   These vary by category, as follows:

Antibiotics. Antibiotics can suppress the immune system as well as diminish sperm production. Exposure to antibiotics may result from consumption of traces in meat, poultry, milk, and prescription drugs.

Anticonvulsants. Anticonvulsants such as phenytoin—Dilantin®—reduce fertility and increase abnormal sperm. Residues are found in the sperm of men taking the drug.

Cancer drugs. Drugs used against malignancies can completely stop sperm production. It may take several years to resume sperm production once therapy ends.

DES (diethylstilbestrol). A synthetic estrogen given to pregnant women during 1941 to 1971, DES has been found to have caused increased genital and sperm abnormalities, infertility, and testicular cancer in male offspring. DES was also frequently added to animal feed until it was banned in 1979.

Ulcer drugs. Cimetidine—Tagamet®—is used for peptic ulcer disease. Ulcer drugs have been shown to reduce sperm count as much as 43 percent after six weeks of therapy. Impotency has also been reported after cimetidine use.

Chemicals

In 1979 a chemistry professor at Florida State University, Robert C. Dougherty, discovered in sperm samples taken from students twenty different chemicals affecting sperm production. Among the chemicals Dougherty found were DDT, benzene compounds, polychlorinated biphenyls (PCBs), and one closely related to the now-banned fireproofing substance Tris (which was used in furniture, bedding, and pajamas during the 1950s and 1960s).

Today nearly sixty thousand chemicals are used in the workplace, but, according to the federal Office of Technology Assessment, fewer than a dozen are regulated to reduce their effects on human reproductive systems.

For example, in a study performed in Quebec, men exposed to hydrocarbons were three times more likely than unexposed men to have had a child die from malignant disease before age five. Exposure to carbon disulfide used in manufacturing viscose rayon has also been linked to sperm abnormalities, reduced sex drive, and increased risk of miscarriage for the exposed workers' wives.

Vinyl chloride, a ubiquitous ingredient found in plastics, can cause chromosomal abnormalities, miscarriage in the wives of exposed workers, reduced sex drive, impotence, neural tube defects, and even neonatal death.

Childhood leukemia has been linked with preconception exposure by the father to chlorinated solvents, spray paints and dyes, methyl ethyl ketone, and cutting oil. Any occupation exposing men to high levels of automobile exhaust has been linked to increased risk of miscarriages.

California's Proposition 65, called the Safe Drinking Water and Toxic Enforcement Act of 1986, provided for the identification of chemicals known to cause reproductive toxicity. See Table 5 for a list of chemicals that have been found to cause functional or structural abnormalities in the male reproductive system.

One chemical that has received widespread publicity is Agent Orange, which was used extensively as a weed killer during the Vietnam War and, more recently, in the United States. Vietnam veterans have complained of numerous health effects due to their exposure to Agent Orange—both in themselves and in their children, including birth defects.

Table 5. Chemicals known to the state of California to cause male reproductive toxicity, as of January 1, 1992 (excluding pharmaceuticals)

Carbon disulfide

Cyclophosphamide (anhydrous)

Cyclophosphamide (hydrated)

1.2-Dibromo-3-chloropropane (DBCP)

Dinitrobenzene

Dinoseb

Ethylene glycol monoethyl ether

Ethylene glycol monomethyl ether

Lead

Tobacco smoke (directly inhaled)

Source: State of California Safe Drinking Water and Toxic Enforcement Act of 1986

It is thought that a byproduct of its manufacturing process, a chemical family called dioxins, are to blame for Agent Orange's effect on health. Although not every study has linked Agent Orange to birth defects, the Centers for Disease Control found Vietnam veterans who were probably exposed to Agent Orange fathered children with spina bifida, cleft lip, congenital cancers, and coloboma (an eye defect) more often than did unexposed men. According to the March of Dimes, the cause-and-effect relationship between Agent Orange exposure and these particular birth defects is still uncertain.

Scientists have not always been able to identify precisely which chemical might be causing a problem, but they have linked specific occupations with increased risk of certain birth defects. Firemen, for example, are known to be at greater than normal risk of producing children with heart defects. The children of bus and truck drivers and mechanics, machinists, miners, and painters seem especially susceptible to leukemia-lymphoma and nervous system malignancies. Children of aircraft industry workers, printers, construction workers, and paper millers have a high incidence of nervous-system tumors.

Radiation

Like women, men may be exposed to radiation through their work, the atmosphere, or medical therapy. The damage inflicted by radiation exposure accumulates over a lifetime.

Men's chronic exposure to ionizing radiation (such as in the medical profession or in nuclear power plants) has been associated with increased frequency of chromosomal abnormalities among aborted fetuses, stillbirths, neural tube defects, childhood leukemia, and very low birth weight. There is also more genetic mutation in sperm.

During the past decade, international research has also accumulated that links men's occupational exposure to nonionizing electromagnetic energy fields (such as work in electrical occupations) and greater likelihood of abnormalities in their young children, including brain cancer or malformations due to chromosomal changes in sperm.

· W H A T   T O   D O ·

☑ Maintaining general good health and sound nutrition can serve as a buffer against environmental pollution. Eating certain nutrients that bind with toxic elements can also help.

Seaweed and garlic, for example, both help the body eliminate lead and mercury. Other nutrients facilitate the liver's ability to detoxify chemicals and drugs and help to produce and maintain strong, healthy sperm. (See "Preconception Care" for details.) Be sure, however, to confer with a nutritionally trained medical professional before using nutritional supplements to treat any medical condition.

☑ If you are offered a prescription drug just before you intend to conceive a child, ask your physician or pharmacist about the drug's effects on reproduction.

☑ Stop smoking cigarettes or marijuana. Avoid inhaling others' cigarette smoke.

☑ Investigate your workplace for potential hazards. Ask yourself: Which substances are you exposed to? At what concentration level? How long are you exposed? (In general, it takes months of exposure to harm sperm production and quality.) Are you frequently splashed with chemicals? Can you see dust, smell odors, or taste vapors? Do you feel lightheaded or have a headache after working in certain areas? Are you provided adequate ventilation and protective gear (worksuits, masks, gloves)? Read "What to Do" at the end of "Occupational Hazards for Women" for further suggestions on investigating the hazards of your workplace.

☑ If you must undergo extensive radiation therapy, consider placing samples of your sperm in a sperm bank before therapy begins. Refrain from attempting to conceive a child until at least ten weeks after therapy ends. After extensive exposure to radiation, it may take even longer for a man's fertility to return to normal.

☑ If you are concerned that you may have genetic damage due to Agent Orange exposure, the March of Dimes can help you locate counseling and testing. The National Information Service (NIS) at the University of South Carolina helps veterans who have children with birth defects and learning disorders find educational, residential, financial, or medical assistance. Call 800-922-9234 (outside South Carolina) or 800-922-1107, extension 401 (inside South Carolina).

PART TWO

During Pregnancy

Prenatal Care

Not until the 1920s did it become common for women in the United States to see a doctor or midwife as soon as they knew they were pregnant and to continue office visits with increasing frequency as the pregnancy progressed. The benefits of prenatal care quickly became evident. Women who receive adequate prenatal care are four times more likely to give birth to a baby with optimal weight who lives and prospers the first year of life than are women who do not receive this care.

Routine examinations of the pregnant woman enable a medical professional to detect emotional and physical problems that might affect the health of the mother or the child, or influence the birth. For example, premature labor, small-for-age babies, maternal infections, anemia, high blood pressure, gestational diabetes, malnutrition, multiple births, or breech presentation may all be discovered early enough to allow proper intervention.

Prenatal care also provides a chance for the pregnant woman to receive help in eliminating unhealthy lifestyle habits, such as skipping meals, eating only refined and nutrition-poor foods, smoking cigarettes, or drinking alcohol. These unhealthy habits can weigh heavily on a scale that is already tipped toward premature delivery due to certain medical conditions, such as carrying more than one fetus, a previous preterm labor, a lax (also called incompetent) cervix, uterine fibroids, an unusually shaped uterus, a history of infertility or in vitro fertilization, abdominal surgery earlier in the pregnancy, a previous cervical cone biopsy, or exposure to DES before the pregnant woman's own birth.

Although medical care is important during pregnancy, nonobstetric surgery may not be a good idea during this time. In 1989 an American-Swedish collaborative study of over five thousand Swedish women who underwent nonobstetrical operations during their pregnancies found a

46 percent increase in the rate of premature deliveries and of infants with very low and low birth weight. In addition, infants whose mothers underwent operations during pregnancy suffered higher infant death rates during the week following birth than infants whose mothers did not have operations. The same study found that after a first trimester operation, regardless of the nature of the operation, women had nearly two and a half times more babies with neural tube defects (NTD) than expected. The researchers noticed that nearly all were operated on during week four or five, which is when the fetal neural tube closes. What isn't clear is whether it was the woman's condition that led to surgery, the trauma of the operation itself, or drugs used during surgery that were involved in these adverse pregnancy outcomes.

· W H A T   T O   D O ·

☑ Go for prenatal care as soon as you know you are pregnant or at least by the time you are three months pregnant.

Obstetricians, family practitioners, and midwives have individual personalities; their approaches to prenatal care and to birth vary widely. Find a medical office that fits your personality and needs. If you and your health provider are properly matched, your trust and respect for each other will buoy you through even the roughest pregnancy and delivery.

☑ Ask if your employer is among the 375 companies offering the March of Dimes prenatal health education program called "Babies and You."

☑ Avoid having surgery during weeks four and five of your pregnancy. If surgery is an emergency, remember that 2252 women in the Swedish study had operations during their first trimester and 2208 had a child with no significant malformations of any kind. The odds are definitely in your favor to give birth to a healthy child, too.

☑ Educate yourself. Today's books on pregnancy include every possible detail of the experience. Here are some of my favorites: *The Well Pregnancy Book*, by Michael and Nancy Samuels; *Childbirth with Love*, by Dr. Niels Lauersen; *Pregnancy and Childbirth*, by Tracy Hotchner; *Woman-Centered Pregnancy and Birth,* by Ginney Cassidy-Brinn, R.N., and others; *What to Expect When You're Expecting,* by Arlene Eisenberg and others; any book by the thoroughly enlightened and enlightening Sheila Kitzinger; and *An Easier Childbirth,* by Gayle Peterson, Ph.D.

———————————————————————————

Prematurity,
Low Birth Weight,
and Stress

E motional stress has long been linked to problems with pregnancy. Even William Shakespeare mentioned in *A Winter's Tale* that "frights and griefs" could lead to premature delivery. Thanks to modern research, we now know that emotional stress can also cause low birth weight.

Premature delivery refers to labor occurring before the end of the 37th week and is often called preterm labor, since full-term babies are born between the 38th and 40th weeks. Some 6 to 8 percent of births (between 250,000 and 400,000 babies) are born prematurely in the United States each year; they account for the majority of deaths or developmental diseases among newborns. For those who survive birth after only a 30-week term, medical costs can become astronomical; some of these babies require lifelong special care. For example, a preterm baby is five times more likely to have cerebral palsy than is a full-term baby.

A full-term baby under 2500 grams (around 5.5 pounds) is considered to have a low birth weight. This condition may be due to preterm delivery or to the baby not developing appropriately in relation to its gestational age. Low birth weight is also a prime cause of infant mortality. The United States has one of the highest rates of low birth weight of any industrialized nation.

The connection between stress and prematurity and low birth weight is both direct and indirect. Emotional stress, itself, can cause these problems. Alternately, behaviors that lead to prematurity and low birth weight—such as the use of cigarettes, alcohol, or cocaine, or undernourishment and poor weight gain—may be in response to the depression and anxiety that accompany such stressful situations as severe financial need or lack of social support. It is not surprising that the babies of low-income women are especially at risk of prematurity and low birth weight.

Some research has suggested that the effect of stress on the fetus is especially acute during the second trimester. In 1989 the *Journal of Family Practice* published a study of 513 women receiving prenatal care at four different family practices in rural America. Major life changes during the second trimester, such as death of a spouse, loss of a job, or a move, were seen to precipitate significantly higher rates of poor pregnancy outcomes—such as neonatal death, transfer to a neonatal intensive-care unit, low birth weight, and relatively lower Apgar scores (which rate a newborn's overall condition).

Further research reported in 1991 from England, Scotland, and Denmark suggests that the second trimester is also an especially vulnerable time for the psychological development of the fetus.

The good news is, whatever your life situation, you may be able to prevent the ill effects of stress. Whether the stress begins during your pregnancy or has built up for years, current research suggests that in some cases it is more important to change your attitude toward the situation than it is to change the situation itself.

For example, an article in the *American Journal of Public Health* (February 1990) suggested it was the pregnant employee's attitude toward her job, including whether she was working by choice or would prefer to be at home, that correlated best with her risk of preterm or low–birth-weight delivery—regardless of the physical labor her job demanded.

STRESS REDUCTION

Lewis E. Mehl, M.D., Ph.D. (now of the Department of Family Practice, University of Vermont) has been able to prevent premature delivery by helping women identify and ease the emotional influences upon premature labor. Mehl, in a provocative article in *Mothering* (Fall 1988) describes five major categories of emotional stress that may precipitate premature labor.

- High levels of family discord and an overwhelming sense of responsibility for the family's well-being. Under hypnosis these women reveal an unconscious belief that an early delivery would allow them to focus on other family members' needs, since hospital nurses would care for the new baby.

- Inability to express extreme anxiety about the pregnancy. Under hypnosis these women reveal an unconscious desire to be cared for at the hospital.

- A perceived need to appear perfectly fine. These women may be unaware of their internal body state. They may have rising blood pressure, but report that everything is fine.

- Fear of delivery. These women may hope a smaller baby will be easier to deliver.

- A history of poor health. These women may be so accustomed to being dependent on health professionals that they unconsciously elicit the need for medical care.

Mehl found that even after preterm labor began, it could be stopped until closer to the proper due date through the use of psychotherapy, bodywork, and biofeedback (a means of learning how to recognize subtle cues from one's nervous system and to use them to alter the body's reactions to stress). In addition, Mehl and his colleagues used family therapy to help the fathers-to-be ease into new roles and responsibilities, which lessened the women's stress in the marital relationship. Hypnosis, by the way, has been reported by American, Soviet, and Israeli researchers to be a useful adjunct to conventional therapy for premature labor.

THE FRENCH MODEL

The cost of the special medical care the preemies receive, which is paid for by both individuals and their insurance companies, adds up to about $5 billion a year. All the expensive equipment and lifesaving techniques regularly used in U.S. hospitals has not significantly reduced the annual number of premature births and babies with low birth weight. Yet, these conditions can be prevented. France has done it without the need to rely on expensive, high-tech solutions; following France's example, several individual programs in California, North Carolina, and Minnesota have reduced the incidence of this category of birth defect.

For twelve years, from 1971 through 1982, Emile Papiernik, M.D., organized the largest contemporary study of perinatal intervention, involving more than sixteen thousand live births in Haguenau, France. During the first three years of the study there were no significant changes in low birth weight or prematurity, as women and their care providers needed to become accustomed to the required changes in lifestyle. But in time, among the population studied, Papiernik was able to reduce the number of premature births by one-third and the number of babies having very low birth weight (less than 3.25 pounds) and very premature infants (born before thirty-four weeks) by two-thirds—except among women at high risk (such as teens and those with previous preterm deliveries).

The French program is the ultimate in common sense: If examination of a woman's cervix indicates changes that suggest a risk of early labor, she is requested to limit her activity level, reduce her stress, and modify her work schedule on doctor's orders—with no loss of pay, as stipulated by French law. Free household help is available through the French social service system if family or friends cannot provide it. A weekly follow-up by a nurse-midwife ensures ongoing communication and professional support.

In the United States, similar results have been reported in a hospital affiliated with the University of California, San Francisco; in a twenty-county region in North Carolina; and in a rural practice in Minnesota. These programs, oriented around patient education, were not only medically successful but also economically advantageous. Financial analysts in North Carolina figured the savings from the program to be $11.27 for every dollar they spent.

· W H A T   T O   D O ·

☑ If you feel stress, try to limit your activity level. Take some time off from your work, if possible. Ask for help from friends and relatives for errands and household tasks.

☑ Immediately report the following signs of premature labor to your health provider: uterine contractions; feelings of pressure, backache, or undefined discomfort in thighs or intestines; diarrhea; or vaginal discharge of blood or mucus.

☑ Change your point of view to reduce your stress. Inevitably, there will be unpleasant circumstances over which you have no control. Instead of being bitter, decide that no matter how many lemons life throws at you, you will make lemonade. Even if you cannot change others, you are in control of your reaction to what others do and say. As research has shown, your attitude is the source of your power.

☑ Get professional advice, if needed. Counselors may be found through county mental-health departments, university health centers, and family service organizations. Low-cost counseling is available through schools offering advanced degrees in social work, counseling, and psychology. Do not forget about local clergy, too. At the very least, confide in a close friend and do some problem solving together.

☑ Get support during stressful times. The more social support a mother receives, the less effect her stress has on her infant. If family and friends are the source of emotional stress, remove yourself from their influence. You may find needed support in a self-help group. Connect with groups in your area by calling The American Self-Help Clearinghouse, 201-625-7101.

☑ Handle any financial problems creatively. Worry about financial problems is associated with an incidence of low birth weight that is six times higher than usual. Instead of believing you are trapped, assume there is a solution and determine to find it. Remember, a belief that you cannot change your feeling of helplessness and hopelessness is more dangerous to your well-being than the prejudice, bad luck, wrong choices, and illnesses you face.

☑ Recognize that your mate may also be under stress. He may be frightened of the enormous responsibility of fatherhood or anxious about the inevitable changes in your relationship and finances. He may turn that anxiety into anger, which is easier to express, or he may withdraw, which feels safer. All of the suggestions above apply equally to men. So, if needed, suggest to him that he, too, learn ways to reduce his stress. To provide for the safety and health of his unborn child, a father-to-be must help create an environment of emotional tranquility within which the entire family can flourish.

☑ You may find special inspiration in the following books:
Love Is Letting Go of Fear, by Gerald Jampolsky, M.D. (Bantam 1989). Jampolsky overcame heavy drinking, back pain, divorce, and depression by changing his attitude and values to those described in this cartoon-rich paperback.
The Dance of Anger: A Woman's Guide to Changing the Patterns of Intimate Relationships, by Harriet Goldhor Lerner,

Ph.D. (Harper & Row 1985). An immensely useful book for every adult woman, showing you how to use your anger (at parent, spouse, child, employer) to your best advantage— especially useful if getting angry has up to now been getting you nowhere.

Getting the Love You Want: A Guide for Couples, by Harville Hendrix, Ph.D. (Henry Holt 1988). If your relationship with your mate is a major cause of stress, this book may be one of the most helpful sources for improvement.

How to Survive Unbearable Stress, by Steven L. Burns, M.D. (I-Med Press 1990). Unpretentious, large type, easy to understand and read, and illustrated with endearing cartoons.

Diet and Nutrition

Nutrition is one of the most important factors determining the outcome of your pregnancy, for what you eat determines in great measure both your health and that of your fetus. You are very lucky that it is almost entirely under your control.

NUTRITIONAL DEFICIENCIES
AND BIRTH DEFECTS

Not too long ago, people believed that the fetus would pull whatever nutrients it needed from the mother's body and so would rarely be affected by nutritional deficiencies. This belief was proven wrong when scientists looked at children born to moderately malnourished Europeans during and just after World War II. They found cardiovascular abnormalities, retarded bone development, neural tube defects, and other anomalies.

Birth defects continue to be caused by inadequate diets and, in particular, insufficient vitamins and minerals. In one study, for example, women whose blood indicated a zinc deficiency early in their pregnancies had abnormal labor, premature or late delivery, underdeveloped infants, and infants with congenital malformations. Women who had had similar low zinc measurements at the beginning of their pregnancy but were supplemented with the mineral had fewer abnormalities.

In 1988 the Centers for Disease Control also revealed that women taking prenatal multivitamins sharply reduced their risk of producing babies with neural tube defects (NTDs). Use of supplements at the time of conception and through the early weeks of pregnancy had the greatest impact. The positive role of nutritional supplements in reducing NTDs has been repeated in studies in Australia, England, and the United States.

NTDs are one of the most frequently encountered categories of central nervous system malformations worldwide; they include anencephaly (absence of the brain) and spina bifida (incomplete closure of the spinal column). Although the incidence of NTDs in the United States has declined since the 1930s (which, significantly, was the era of widespread belt-tightening called The Great Depression), approximately three thousand infants are born each year with potentially lethal, sometimes paralyzing NTDs.

Another study of the relationship between prenatal multivitamins and birth defects was published in 1982 in the *Lancet* (a British medical journal). Czechoslovakian women who had already delivered a child with a cleft lip or cleft palate were provided low-dose multivitamins during the three months before and the three months after conception. Cleft rates in their children were around 1 percent, compared to around 7 percent for children of a comparable group who were not given vitamin supplements.

The Unaware Eater

Even if you are eating regular meals each day, you and your fetus still may be inadequately nourished. Some explanations for this follow:

- In 1991 the Food and Drug Administration conducted the Total Diet Study and found insufficient amounts of calcium, magnesium, iron, and zinc in the diets of adult American women. Eating three meals or more a day does not help if they contain large quantities of products having white flour and white sugar, which lack many of the vitamins, minerals, and enzymes found in fresh produce, seeds, and whole grains.

- The Recommended Dietary Allowance (RDA) for each nutrient is only a baseline figure, created by statistical analysis of the amount of vitamins needed to prevent the grossest symptoms of vitamin deficiency in the average healthy person. There is, however, no average person. The nutrient requirements of individuals can vary tenfold or more due to genetic differences. Several studies have suggested that the mothers of children with NTDs may have a genetic need for more than the usual level of folic acid and zinc in their diets.

  Marginal deficiencies are usually not noticed. Well before diseases like scurvy (vitamin C deficiency) or beri-beri (vitamin B deficiency) appear, marginal deficiencies may occur and cause symptoms, such as irritability, fatigue, depression, mood shifts, chest pains, muscle cramps, diarrhea alternating with constipation, headaches, recurrent colds, difficulty concentrating, or poor memory.

- Even a diet of fresh produce may contain less nutrition than you think, since farmland differs and may be naturally high or low in particular minerals. For example, a carrot from Maryland may contain 1.8 micrograms of selenium, while a carrot from South Dakota may contain 105.3 micrograms of the mineral.

- Nutrients are lost when food is stored, processed, heated, packaged, preserved, and cooked in excess water or high heat. For example, people who eat white bread are missing 70 to 80 percent of the B-1, B-2, B-3, and B-6 found in whole wheat bread. Moreover, so much vitamin B complex and minerals are leached out of vegetables and legumes when boiled that you are better off throwing away the food and drinking the cooking water.

- Chronic infections, diseases, allergies, and other medical conditions can strip the body of nutrients and cause poor absorption of those consumed. Even pharmaceuticals may deplete the body of nutrients. For example, aspirin reduces the body's levels of folic acid, vitamin C, and iron.

- Bad habits also take their nutritional toll: Every cigarette you smoke uses up 250 mg of your body's vitamin C plus some folic acid, thiamine, and calcium. The caffeine in coffee reduces vitamin B complex, vitamin C, zinc, potassium, and inositol.

- Millions of women habitually restrict their diet in order to lose weight, thus reducing their intake of essential nutrients even more than usual.

- Salt is often unrecognized for its role in maintaining a healthy pregnancy. In 1958 Dr. Margaret Robinson of St. Thomas Hospital, London, reported in the *Lancet* her comparison of the outcome of pregnancy between groups using or avoiding salt. Her study is old but important, since her experimentation on human subjects would never be allowed today. She found more abnormal placentas, two and a half times as many cases of pre-eclamptic toxemia (a potentially life-threatening condition), and twice as many infants dying around the time of birth among a thousand pregnant women who followed orders to eat a low-salt diet during pregnancy, compared to a thousand pregnant women who were ordered to eat a relatively high salt diet.

In sum, international research has revealed direct connections between a successful pregnancy and improved nutrition, including supplementation of multivitamins and minerals. Again, this is one area in which you have total control. By choosing wholesome foods for every meal, you are giving yourself the best chance for a successful pregnancy and a healthy child.

· W H A T   T O   D O ·

☑ To ensure nutritionally adequate meals, do your best to eat the colors of the rainbow in your food every day: purple cabbage, green leafy vegetables (folic acid derives its name from foliage), red beets or strawberries, and so on. Your daily rainbow of food might contain the white of dairy, since dairy products are a good source of calcium. Milk, however, is not the only source of calcium: There is actually more in a cup of garbanzo beans (300 mg), salmon (339 mg), sardines (375 mg per can), or almonds (304 mg) than in a cup of milk (288 mg).

☑ Although raw meat or raw fish may have been an enjoyable part of your diet in the past, these foods ought to be avoided during the months of pregnancy. See the section on toxoplasmosis in "Infectious Diseases" for more information on this issue.

☑ Make eating well easy: Keep vegetables crisp in a container of water in the refrigerator for quick snacks. Munch air-popped popcorn instead of greasy chips or sweets while you watch television.

☑ Salt your food to taste.

☑ Use red raspberry leaf tea as a daily drink during pregnancy. Red raspberry leaves contain fragine (which helps produce effective contractions and an easier labor), iron, calcium, and magnesium—which are all needed in increasing amounts during pregnancy. The herb can be combined with peppermint and honey for flavor. Steep a teaspoon of each herb in a quart of water for a few minutes, then strain and sip throughout the day.

☑ Consult with your doctor about taking a prenatal vitamin formula that is right for you. (If you have epilepsy, check with your doctor about possible folic acid–anticonvulsant interactions.) If the vitamin formula also contains minerals, be sure the directions call for taking several tablets a day. If you are only supposed to take one tablet a day, you will probably be consuming a very minor amount of minerals.

Note: There is no guarantee that supplementing your diet with folic acid, zinc, or the full complement of prenatal vitamins and minerals will necessarily prevent the birth of a child with spina bifida, cleft lip, or any other birth defect. Yet, knowing that spina bifida rates drop dramatically with preconception vitamin and mineral supplementation, why not provide yourself the preventive measure of a commercially prepared prenatal formula, which may cost about $22 a month?

☑ Avoid excessive use of individual supplements, especially vitamin A. Birth defects have occurred when women used high doses of vitamin A (over 20,000 IU daily) or continued to consume Accutane, a vitamin A derivative prescribed for severe acne, while pregnant.

☑ If needed, pregnant women can obtain vouchers from their local Department of Public Social Service that allow them to purchase nutritious food through the Special Supplemental Food Program for Women, Infants, and Children (WIC).

☑ You may wish to obtain professional dietary advice from someone licensed to provide nutritional counseling. In one study, women receiving such counseling prior to pregnancy gained six pounds more weight and delivered a third fewer infants with low birth weight than did those not counseled. One source of referrals is the American Dietetic Association, 216 West Jackson Boulevard, Chicago, Ill. 60606-6995, 312-899-0040, extension 4815. Or, look in the Yellow Pages of your phone book for physicians trained in nutrition. You may also obtain local referrals for medical doctors knowledgeable in nutrition from the American Holistic Medical Association, 4101 Lake Boone Trail, Suite 201, Raleigh, N.C. 27607, 919-787-5146; and the Price-Pottenger Nutrition Foundation, 5871 El Cajon Boulevard, San Diego, Calif. 92115, 619-582-4168.

☑ Read *What Every Pregnant Woman Should Know,* by Gail S.
Brewer (Penguin 1985); *Total Nutrition During Pregnancy,* by
Betty Kamen, Ph.D., and Si Kamen (Keats 1986); and *Wise-
Woman Herbal for the Childbearing Year,* by Susun Weed (Ash
Tree Publishing 1986).

A NOTE ABOUT DIETING
DURING PREGNANCY

Some women become unduly concerned about their weight during pregnancy. They and their spouse view the woman's growing belly with a mixture of pleasure and alarm. It is imperative that you do not attempt to lose
weight immediately before or during pregnancy. Resulting nutritional deficiencies may be devastating for the child you conceive, for the following
reasons:

- Dieting before pregnancy increases the risk of perinatal death and
  birth defects.

- Dieting during pregnancy threatens the fetus with brain damage or
  low birth weight, putting the infant at risk of serious complications,
  hospitalization, and neonatal death.

- Numerous studies have found that underweight women produce more
  babies of low birth weight, more babies born before term, and more
  babies with anemia, cardiac and respiratory problems, and low Apgar scores.

In 1990 the National Academy of Science's Subcommittee on Nutritional Status and Weight Gain During Pregnancy was asked to recommend figures indicating healthy levels of weight gain. The subcommittee
found that women of normal weight for their height who are carrying one
fetus have the best chance of preventing low birth weight when they gain
25 to 35 pounds.

Average-weight newborns are regularly delivered by women who gain
only 16 pounds—and by those who gain 40 pounds or more. The range is
wide, indicating that the mother's weight gain is not the only factor determining birth weight. What you consume is ultimately more important
than the quantity consumed. Once you become pregnant you are in the
baby construction business, and every mouthful you eat is part of another
day's work. Use superior materials to get the job done the best way you can.

· W H A T   T O   D O ·

☑ Be sensitive to your body's desire for food. During pregnancy your desire for food may alter, and you may have strong and unexplained cravings. Your senses heighten, and certain common food odors may now be unbearable. Your blood volume increases; your heart beats faster; and your temperature rises, making hot foods less appealing. Edema, a swelling that results from excess fluid in connective tissue, is normal but adds to your feeling of bulkiness. Late in pregnancy, in addition to increased edema, you may feel sluggish due to slowed digestion. Muscles relax, including the sphincter between your stomach and esophagus, so you may experience uncomfortable feelings of heartburn and acidity. For all these reasons, you may not be consuming your usual variety or quantity of food. At this time, more than ever, you need to pay special attention to eating well.

☑ If you were of average weight at the beginning of pregnancy, you should be gaining around 1 pound per week during your second and third trimesters. If you begin pregnancy thin, try to gain a little more than a pound a week, and if you began greatly overweight, you can gain less than a pound a week and remain within the recommended range.

☑ Ask for the scientific basis of any recommendations your health-care practitioner may make to restrict your weight, reduce your salt, or treat your edema with diuretics.

☑ Start noticing that pregnant women are beautiful. Their faces need little makeup to glow, because extra blood is so close to the surface of the skin. The natural edema of pregnancy makes wrinkles disappear. If you are currently pregnant, look in the mirror and rejoice. This is no time to diet. It is, however, a time to avoid the empty calories of convenience and junk foods. Instead, fill your plate with the foods of high nutritional quality: grains, beans, vegetables, dairy products, nuts, seeds, fruits, poultry, fish, and red meats.

Prescription and Over-the-Counter Drugs

After nutrition, pharmaceutical drugs are the most important area of concern for pregnant women. Medications are thought to account for anywhere from less than 1 percent to 10 percent of birth defects. In a study by Bracken and Holford in Connecticut investigating the effects of pharmaceuticals during all three trimesters of pregnancy, the use of any prescribed drug, on the average, raised a woman's risk of a birth defect by 30 percent. The risk was especially high with specific drugs, like Valium, or if a woman also smoked cigarettes. Since the cause of about 70 percent of birth defects is still unknown, it is possible that future research will prove pharmaceuticals to be an even greater influence on birth defects.

Many medications can pass across the placenta by simple diffusion, reaching levels in a baby's blood from 10 to 100 percent of that in the mother's blood. For various biochemical reasons, some medicines are found in the fetal bloodstream at even greater concentrations than in the bloodstream of the mother.

Medicines pose the most risk of creating physical malformations from the second to eighth weeks after conception. During these weeks of major organ formation, each cell has enormous influence on the future development of body structures. Exposure to one hazardous drug may cause several different malformations, especially if the embryo is exposed while simultaneously developing several different limbs and organs. Even at the end of pregnancy, cells in the ear, eye, sex organs, liver, and brain are dividing rapidly and are vulnerable to damage by pharmaceuticals.

Not every medication, however, causes malformations. Although over six hundred pharmaceuticals can cause malformations in animals, fewer than twenty-five are recognized as teratogens that cause physical damage in human beings (see Table 6). Therefore, never make a hasty decision about terminating a pregnancy simply because a medicine you took appears on a list of teratogens. No teratogenic medication has ever produced birth defects in the children of every single woman who took it. The effects of any drug depend on many factors, including dose and timing of consumption. Discuss your concerns about a medicine's toxicity with your physician and pharmacist. Other sources, such as pregnancy exposure hotlines for free and fast counseling, are listed in Appendix B.

Pharmaceuticals have many other possible effects besides malformations. They can alter the unborn baby's growth or cause functional problems where organs are well-formed but do not work correctly, miscarriages, cancer in childhood or adulthood, mental retardation, learning difficulties, or mutations that, if they occur in a sex cell, may be passed on to future generations.

Table 6. Selected Drugs Teratogenic in Humans (in decreasing risk of teratogenicity)

Generic Drug (one common brand)	Most common defects observed	Risk of defect (percent)
anticonvulsant: Trimethadione (Tridione®)	facial abnormalities, congenital heart disease, growth retardation, mental retardation, genital defects	60
anticancer: Aminopterin	neural tube defects, oral clefts, limb defects	30
female hormone: Diethylstilbestrol (DES)	uterine and cervical abnormalities, testicular abnormalities, minute penis, vaginal cancer	22–58
dermatological: Isotretinoin (Accutane®)	central nervous system abnormalities, ear absence or abnormalities, heart defects, thymus gland defect	20
androgenic hormone: testosterone, progestins	masculinization of female genitals	0.3–18

Unfortunately, whether or not your use of medication will harm your baby is difficult to predict. The potential for damage depends not only on the type of drug taken but also on the metabolism of the mother, genetic predispositions in the mother and fetus, the health of their livers (the major detoxifying organ) and kidneys (the body's filtration center), and the stage of development of the fetus.

A woman's state of health and level of stress can affect how much of a pharmaceutical transfers to the fetus. Once transferred, the ability to repair drug damage can be influenced by the nutritional status of the fetus's body tissues. Other important factors include the dose, the week of pregnancy, and even the time of day a pharmaceutical is taken. Since our body has what is called a circadian rhythm (which changes our metabolism according to a species-specific biological clock) these rhythms influence

Table 6. (Continued)

Generic Drug (one common brand)	Most common defects observed	Risk of defect (percent)
anti-cancer: Other than aminopterin	depends on drug	over all 17
tranquilizer: Lithium (Eskalith®)	congenital heart defects	11
anticonvulsant: Phenytoin (Dilantin®)	abnormal fingertips and nails, abnormal facial features, deficient growth	10
anticoagulant: Coumarin (Warfarin®)	abnormal nose, mental retardation, congenital heart disease	7
anticonvulsant: Valproic acid	spina bifida	1

Adapted from Stanley, F.J., and C. Bower. "Teratogenic Drugs in Pregnancy." *The Medical Journal of Australia* 1986, 145:596–99 (Table 2). Copyright 1986 *The Medical Journal of Australia*, reprinted with permission.

drug effectiveness. Thus, the same dose of aspirin taken first thing in the morning delivers a greater dose to the bloodstream than at bedtime. An antacid taken at night can be two or three times as effective as the same dose taken in the morning.

The length of time it takes to assess a medicine's effect on birth defects complicates the analysis. Pediatricians and child psychiatrists often do not ask about obstetric drug history when consulted about a child's learning disabilities, short attention span, or physical difficulties. So we have limited knowledge about the connections between medications and many long-term problems.

Ultimately, every pregnant woman taking a medication is a unique universe in which that drug acts. Medical ethics forbids testing drugs on pregnant women, so a drug's potential effect for each woman is usually unknown and may only reveal itself over time—as physicians and patients begin to associate medication use with certain defects or problems.

The following is a brief review of some reproductive effects of common prescription drugs, alphabetically listed by use or generic name. Brand names may be given in parentheses or separated by dashes. Be sure you know the generic name of any drug you take. One generic drug may be sold under several different brand names:

Antibiotics and other anti-infectives can often be taken without danger of damaging the fetus, but there are a few that need special caution; check with your physician or pharmacist before consuming any in this category. For example, sulfonamides—also called sulfa drugs, such as Bactrim®, Gantrisin®, and Septra®—have been suspected of causing birth defects, but this association has never been proven.

Two dangerous effects of sulfonamides, however, are generally recognized. One is the possibility of hemolytic anemia in infants with a rare inherited metabolic condition called G6PD deficiency. The other is the danger to newborns who are given sulfonamides of increasing their bilirubin (an orange or yellow bile pigment found in the blood) to the point of developing kernicterus, which is a kind of jaundice that can lead to brain damage. To be extra safe, physicians usually avoid prescribing sulfonamides during the third trimester.

Anticancer drugs, such as methotrexate and aminopterin, cause abortion or, in as many as 30 percent of surviving fetuses, growth delay and deformities of the skull and gonads—probably because they diminish folic acid levels in the body.

Antidepressants, such as amitriptyline (Elavil®), are to be avoided, as some physicians have reported birth defects, including abnormal limbs and cleft palate among infants exposed to this category of drug prenatally.

Antiepileptics may increase the risk of birth defects, including abnormal face and limbs. Also common is a blood coagulation defect leading to hemorrhage in the newborn, which can be prevented with vitamin K injections for you during pregnancy and labor and for your baby after birth. Some research links the father's use of phenytoin to higher rate of birth defects in children.

Since common anticonvulsants can reduce folic acid levels and since deficiency of this B vitamin is associated with birth defects, it may be useful for women planning to become pregnant to have their nutritional status tested and supplemented where necessary (see the section on epilepsy in "Pre-existing Medical Conditions").

Anti-inflammatories, such as cortisone and other corticosteroids (hormones often used to reduce inflammation and to prevent brain edema in cases of trauma), are controversial; one study indicated increased fetal distress and death, another study did not show these effects. At present, low doses (the equivalent of 25 mg per day of cortisone or 5 mg per day of prednisone) are not considered dangerous to the fetus. Corticosteroids can cause calcium loss and some can cause salt and water retention and increase blood pressure, so the pregnant woman's diet may need adjustment.

Nonsteroidal anti-inflammatories, such as ketoprofen (Orudis®) and naproxen (Naprosyn®, Anaprox®), can cause excessive bleeding in the mother and newborn and should be avoided during the last three months of pregnancy.

Acne medications can be dangerous if they contain isotretinoin (Accutane®). At least fifty thousand women of child-bearing age use Accutane® each year in the United States, even though it is a proven teratogen. Major malformations of the ears, skull, palate, and heart, or miscarriages occur in about 20 percent of exposed fetuses. Already, several hundred cases of serious birth defects have occurred in this country due to injected or oral doses of Accutane®.

If you were taking Accutane® but stopped at least one to two months before you conceived, the drug will probably have been eliminated from your body before it could cause any harm to your fetus. The critical period of exposure is from the fourth to the tenth weeks after conception, which includes weeks you may not know you are pregnant. Do not donate blood while you are using Accutane® or you may pass the drug on to someone else during her early months of pregnancy.

Some high blood pressure medications can cause birth defects of the face and limbs, problems with the lungs and kidneys, and even death if women are exposed during their second or third trimesters of pregnancy. The dangerous medications belong to a class of drugs called angiotensin-converting enzyme inhibitors, or ACE inhibitors. According to the FDA, women on ACE inhibitors should inform their physician and switch to less dangerous drugs to control their blood pressure, or seek alternative treatment.

Psoriasis is an uncomfortable and unsightly skin condition often treated with etretinate—Tegison®—a known teratogen. This drug has been found in women's bloodstreams nearly three years following the conclusion of treatment. If you are considering having a child within the next few years, definitely handle your psoriasis with an alternative therapy.

Sedatives are among the most prescribed drugs in the world, used to treat sleep disorders and to help people handle unpleasant moods. They have been used widely during pregnancy to reduce anxiety, increase muscular relaxation, reduce duration of labor, and treat pre-eclampsia and eclampsia. Yet, at least three studies have identified diazepam—Valium®—as a possible teratogen, causing oral clefts when consumed during early pregnancy. Hypothermia (loss of body heat) at birth has also been associated with this drug. When doses greater than 30 mg were given to mothers during labor, symptoms in the newborn included low Apgar scores, stopping of breathing, reluctance to feed, abnormal heartbeats, and reduced muscle tone.

Vaccines that are live, attenuated virus vaccines (such as measles) are not to be used during pregnancy, because of the theoretical possibility that the fetus might develop the disease. The Immunization Advisory Committee at the American College of Obstetricians and Gynecologists suggests using the inactivated polio vaccine only when there is increased risk of exposure to the disease.

OVER-THE-COUNTER DRUGS

In truth, the only safe drug is an ineffective drug. So ask a pharmacist and your physician before consuming any pharmaceutical—even common over-the-counter varieties. Pay attention to any warnings in the package insert about drug-to-drug, or drug-to-food interactions. Remember, unusually high doses of vitamins are not a good idea during pregnancy, either.

Specific Drugs

The following is a brief review of some reproductive effects of common over-the-counter drugs:

Acetaminophen—Tylenol®—is often used to replace aspirin during pregnancy because it is reputedly safer. In one study of children's intelligence during their preschool years, children exposed to acetaminophen in the womb scored better than those exposed to aspirin. Some researchers, however, have suggested that there is not enough data to conclude that acetaminophen is safer than aspirin during pregnancy.

Aspartame is a sweetener used widely in diet drinks and desserts under the trade name NutraSweet® or as the sugar substitute Equal®. It is broken down in the intestine to methanol and two amino acids: phenylalanine and aspartic acid. It is generally considered safe for pregnant women, although allergic reactions to it are also common. Consequently, if you have headaches, symptoms of bladder infection, or other health concerns and are regularly consuming diet drinks, see if your symptoms disappear after eliminating the diet drinks for a week or two. Women with the condition called PKU (phenylketonuria) who must avoid overeating phenylalanine-containing foods need to know that aspartame is a source of this amino acid.

Saccharine—used, for example, in the sugar substitute Sweet 'N Low®—is derived from naphthalene (a derivative of coal tar, a potential carcinogen in animals and frequently the cause of allergic reactions in humans). Saccharine has been marketed in America for over ninety years, yet there is little research on its safety for pregnant women. Exposure before birth could possibly have a more harmful effect than after birth, since the fetus collects the chemical in its tissues to a much greater extent than do adults. Consequently, experts recommend that pregnant women avoid foods sweetened with saccharine.

Aspirin is a controversial drug; some studies indicate that children exposed in utero suffered loss of IQ; some indicate increased risk of oral cleft; and others show neither of these effects. Aspirin is still considered a safe drug in ordinary doses, taken only when really necessary. There is a risk of internal bleeding in infants and mothers. In addition, aspirin may delay the onset of labor and then, once it begins, prolong it. To be extra safe, the drug is not recommended during the last three months of pregnancy.

Diet pills often contain phenylpropanolamine, a stimulant that has been linked to birth defects. Use of phenylpropanolamine during the first trimester has been associated with hypospadias (abnormal opening along the penis) and cataracts. Use of the chemical any time during pregnancy is not advised. Other reported problems after phenylpropanolamine use include dislocation of the hip, pectus excavatum (abnormally depressed area of the chest bone), polydactyly (abnormal number of fingers or toes), and abnormalities of the eye or ear.

Ibuprofen—Advil®, Motrin®—is a nonsteroidal anti-inflammatory that should not be used during the last three months of pregnancy, due to the same potential danger of excessive bleeding in mother and newborn as found with aspirin.

As Raja W. Abdul-Karim notes in *Drugs During Pregnancy*, a balance must be found between prescribing a drug that may harm the fetus and denying a pregnant woman an indicated medication that, if it is not given, may lead to harm for her. "In the last analysis," says Abdul-Karim, "it is the well-informed patient who makes the choice."

· W H A T   T O   D O ·

☑ Consider your pregnancy a "drug-free holiday" and avoid all medication during pregnancy, unless required to preserve your life. If you might become pregnant while taking a prescribed drug, or know you are already pregnant, ask your physician whether the drug will merely mask a temporary discomfort, such as morning sickness, or is needed to cure a medical condition that is dangerous to you or your unborn baby. Headaches, insomnia, morning sickness, respiratory infections, and many other common conditions are often treated equally well with the so-called tincture of time.

☑ Usually, medication with potentially undesirable side effects can be replaced with a different drug. For example, if you must take an anticoagulant, coumadin (Warfarin®), which is dangerous, can be replaced by self-administered heparin, which is not as harmful during pregnancy.

☑ Consider using homeopathic remedies, which are nontoxic, diluted substances that stimulate the body's own healing powers. Remedies are inexpensive, gentle, and effective during pregnancy and for infants and children. In fact, there are no known side effects of homeopathic remedies for pregnant or laboring women. Homeopathic remedies are sold over-the-counter in health-food stores, specialized pharmacies, or by mail-order outlets. In 1991 the *British Medical Journal* published a review of worldwide clinical research on homeopathic medicine and found 81 out of 107 studies revealed positive results. You can order guidebooks and remedies from Homeopathic Educational Services, 2124 Kittredge Street, Berkeley, Calif. 94704, 510-649-0294.

☑ If morning sickness is your problem, know that it is actually a healthy sign that your pregnancy is progressing well. Women with nausea and vomiting during their first trimester have been found less likely to suffer miscarriages or stillbirths and gave birth to fewer premature babies than women without this unpleasant condition. Happily, a recent controlled study has demonstrated significant relief from powdered ginger, even for women so severely affected they were hospitalized. You can purchase ginger capsules in a health-food store or simply drop a slice of raw ginger in a cup of hot water and sip the fragrant tea for relief. There are no reports of harm to mothers or infants from ginger.

☑ Another common reason for taking medication during pregnancy is chronic pain. Look for the cause and eliminate it instead of continually treating the symptom. Consider the possibility that the cause may be something simple that you have overlooked, such as food sensitivity, a high desk or improperly placed computer screen causing muscle contraction while you type, a person in your life who is "a pain in the neck," or maybe a reaction to vapors from cleaning solvents or the outgassing of a new rug or furniture.

☑ For a fee, the following service providers will send reports detailing medical research on many conditions and the most successful treatments: Planetree Health Resource Center, 2040 Webster Street, San Francisco, Calif. 94115, 415-923-3680; The Health Resource, 209 Katherine Drive, Conway, Ark. 72032, 501-329-5272; The World Research Foundation, 15300 Ventura Boulevard, Apartment 405, Sherman Oaks, Calif. 91403, 818-907-5483.

☑ There are several important reference books to help you decide what to do, including the following:

Peace of Mind During Pregnancy, by Christine Kelley-Buchanan (Facts On File 1988): a well-balanced and concise description of the danger or safety of a wide variety of common drugs and chemicals.

Physician's Desk Reference (updated yearly). Ask your physician or pharmacist to see their copy of this compendium of statements submitted by manufacturers on the uses and contraindications for their prescription drugs.

Catalog of Teratogenic Agents, by Thomas H. Shepard, M.D. (The Johns Hopkins University Press 1989): lists research suggesting the danger or safety of 1200 different chemicals and pharmaceuticals. Look for it in a medical library or at your obstetrician's office.

Look in Appendix B for state hotlines that can also provide you with information on medications.

Ask your physician and pharmacist for help finding safer alternatives to drugs or safer doses of required drugs.

Recreational Drugs

At least 10 percent of all babies in the United States are born to mothers who are addicted to alcohol or other recreational drugs. This chapter summarizes the effect of recreational drugs on your baby's health.

Keep in mind that whatever may push you to drink, smoke, or use drugs—such as feelings of anxiety, depression, fear, exhaustion, boredom, or shame—will continue to exist throughout pregnancy and after delivery. The solution is not simply to cease taking toxic drugs but to handle these very legitimate feelings in a way that does not endanger your or your unborn child's health.

ALCOHOL

Alcohol is the leading known cause of mental retardation in the United States, ahead of Down syndrome and spina bifida. It is also the most preventable cause of birth defects.

In 1967 a French family practitioner named Alexandre Lamache described to members of the French Academy of Medicine the results of thirty-seven years of observing his patients. He found that alcohol consumption by mothers and fathers was linked to mental retardation, behavioral disorders, genital malformations, abnormal facial features, neurological defects, and higher-than-normal levels of infant deaths. Soon, others reported similar observations, and by 1973 fetal alcohol syndrome had become a medically recognized cluster of abnormalities. Fetal alcohol syndrome is now diagnosed in about 1 out of every 750 births in the United States.

To be counted as fetal alcohol syndrome, a child's signs and symptoms must include growth retardation before or after birth; abnormalities of the central nervous system, such as abnormal muscle tone, shaking, hyperactivity, poor attention span, or obvious mental retardation; and any two of the facial features that are common with this syndrome: narrow eye width, thin upper lip, underdevelopment of the middle of the face, short upturned nose, and underdeveloped groove between the nose and upper lip. Children with fetal alcohol syndrome have an average IQ of 68 to 70 (with 100 being normal). Even those with normal intelligence commonly develop learning disabilities, speech and language problems, hyperactivity, delayed reaction time, and poor motor coordination. In one study, multiple abnormalities were present in 20 percent of the offspring of heavy alcohol users. Children of even moderate drinkers have been found to be hyperactive.

Pregnant women who drink alcohol increase their risk of spontaneous abortion, infertility, nutritional deficiencies, and more complications during childbirth.

How much alcohol is needed to cause fetal alcohol syndrome? The risk rises as the number of daily drinks increases beyond one per day. However, just one drink a day can cause low birth weight. Note this is per day—not one drink during nine months of pregnancy.

Even Dads may contribute to the problem. Research links a father's heavy drinking during the weeks before conception with learning disabilities in their children. More than 75 percent of children with fetal alcohol syndrome have alcoholic fathers in addition to mothers who drink. Scientists suspect that fathers are the cause of at least some alcohol-related birth defects.

· W H A T   T O   D O ·

☑ Avoid alcohol during the nine months of your pregnancy, including social drinks and even over-the-counter cold remedies containing alcohol. Fill your glass at social occasions with sparkling water and a twist of lemon and when offered alcohol simply repeat No, thank you without apologies or explanations. Don't get caught in the just-this-once trap.

☑ If necessary, get professional help to eliminate the factors causing you to drink or to stop your addiction. Attend Alcoholics Anonymous meetings (search for one for nonsmokers to avoid inhaling others' smoke). Also consider acupuncture:

Medical studies have found acupuncture can successfully eliminate the shakes and other withdrawal symptoms during alcohol detoxification. For programs or practitioners near you, check the yellow pages of your phone book or contact the National Acupuncture Detoxification Association, 3115 Broadway, Apartment 51, New York, N.Y. 10027, 212-993-3100.

☑ If you have been drinking regularly before pregnancy, be sure to take prenatal vitamin and mineral supplements and to eat several helpings of foods rich in folic acid, such as green leafy vegetables, kidney beans, broccoli, cauliflower, orange juice, cantaloupe, green peas, and sweet potatoes. Animal research suggests that folic acid deficiency may be instrumental in the development of fetal alcohol syndrome.

COFFEE AND TEA

No one has proven a direct link between malformations and caffeine, but recent research has correlated caffeine consumption to increased risk of miscarriage and infertility. In 1986 a research team at Yale University conducted a study of caffeine consumption by more than thirty-three thousand pregnant women. It revealed a link between daily consumption of 150 mg of caffeine and a higher risk of miscarriage during the late first or second trimester. (One 5-ounce cup of drip-brewed coffee can contain 110 to 150 mg of caffeine. One 5-ounce cup of tea, brewed five minutes, can contain 20 to 50 mg.)

Coffee and caffeinated-tea consumption definitely affects the nutritional status of the pregnant woman. Caffeine reduces levels of not only vitamin B complex and vitamin C but also calcium, zinc, potassium, magnesium, sodium, and chloride. Caffeine is not the only nutritional hazard in coffee. Certain binding substances found in coffee and tea, called polyphenols, decrease the body's absorption of iron, a mineral often deficient in pregnant women. These polyphenols are found in decaffeinated coffee as well.

Caffeine is a powerful stimulant to the nervous system. It crosses the placenta and reaches the fetus in the same concentration as in the mother's blood. So, when you are feeling tired, irritable, and headachy due to caffeine withdrawal, your unborn baby may be experiencing similar reactions to your addiction.

· W H A T   T O   D O ·

☑ Eliminate caffeine from your diet or reduce your intake significantly. If you are committed to this goal but suffer withdrawal symptoms, try gradually mixing an increased percentage of decaffeinated beverage with your regular drink
until you have totally replaced one with the other. Eventually
switch from decaffeinated coffee to one of the coffee substitutes, such as Cafix, Pero, Dacopa (available in natural
foods stores), or Postum (available in major supermarkets).

☑ Watch out for hidden caffeine. There is as much caffeine in
an Excedrin® tablet (130 mg) as in a cup of coffee, and a
standard dose of Anacin® packs more caffeine (64 mg) than
a regular cola drink (30 to 46 mg). The stimulant NoDoz®
and the weight-control aid Dexatrim® each contain 200 mg
of caffeine. Cafergot®, for migraine headaches, contains
100 mg, and a normal dose of the decongestant Dristan® has
32 mg. Significant doses of caffeine are also found in Pepsi,
Dr. Pepper, Mountain Dew, and Tab.

☑ If you fear being constipated without caffeine, increase
whole grains, fruits, and salads—and do yoga. Yoga will also
help if you have needed a pick-me-up to start the day.

LSD, MARIJUANA, HEROIN, AND COCAINE

Babies born to women who used narcotics during pregnancy may experience withdrawal symptoms for weeks after birth. They screech, have difficulty sleeping, and have difficulty being comforted by the usual hugs and
caresses given to newborns. Years later, they exhibit such problems as hyperactivity and an abnormally brief attention span.

Drug use during pregnancy is no longer a private affair. Authorities
have already slapped criminal charges on drug abusers (including at least
one lawyer) whose babies were born with drugs in their bloodstream.

The following is a brief description of what is known about the effects
of LSD, marijuana, heroin, and cocaine on pregnancy. Be aware that

street drugs are likely to be contaminated with unknown chemicals and that marijuana plants are often sprayed with pesticides, so it is difficult for researchers to separate the effect of any one drug apart from its contaminants.

LSD: Lysergic acid does not seem to cause either chromosomal damage or structural abnormalities; long-term effects on human infants, however, are unknown.

Marijuana: Less than a decade ago, studies indicated as many as 14 percent of pregnant women were indulging in marijuana. The drug crosses the placenta. During labor, it increases the vigor of contractions. Chronic marijuana use during pregnancy is associated with prematurity and behavioral abnormalities, but it does not seem to cause malformations among the infants of heavy users (more than five marijuana cigarettes a week). Behavioral abnormalities evened out to normal by the time the infants reached one year of age.

Cocaine: Due to their mothers' addiction, babies of cocaine users often have damaged nervous systems and learning disabilities.

Cocaine use during the first three months of pregnancy increases birth defects of the urinary tract. Use during the second and third trimesters can cause separation of the placenta from the uterine wall, often leading to premature birth. Placental separation can also cause fetal death or brain damage. Some cocaine-exposed fetuses suffer strokes (localized destruction of brain tissue) before birth.

Heroin and methadone: Approximately 6000 to 9000 babies per year are born to women addicted to heroin or methadone. That makes the incidence of opiate-addicted newborns about equal to those suffering fetal alcohol syndrome.

A female heroin addict has three times the risk of stillbirth as does a nonaddict and a higher incidence of medical complications during pregnancy: including toxemia, infectious diseases, and malnutrition.

The addict's baby has four times the risk of prematurity and six times the risk of inadequate growth as do the infants of nonaddicts, may be born with a smaller head than normal, and is at greater risk of respiratory distress, low birth weight, small size, and neonatal death. Born addicted, the newborn must also endure withdrawal.

There is no documented proof of congenital defects due to heroin or methadone use, although incidences of heart defects and hernias—plus an increased incidence of sudden infant death syndrome—have been reported. Chromosomal aberrations in infants exposed to heroin (but not methadone) have also been found. Symptoms of withdrawal continue in these infants for up to six months after birth, including hyperexcitability, irritability, tremors, sweating, vomiting, abnormally long stretches of wakefulness, impaired sucking, and a marked inability to process information and react appropriately.

At one year of age, heroin-exposed children exhibit disturbed attention span, hyperactivity, delayed fine motor skills, and abnormal muscle tone.

· W H A T   T O   D O ·

☑ Do not use drugs and do not think of them as recreational. Seek help, perhaps from a 12-Step program that offers re-direction and emotional support as you break old patterns and gain the self-confidence to face your moments of stress or emotional lows without the crutch of a drug high. You will find such programs in your local phone book, under either Narcotics or the name of the drug.

☑ Consider learning new stress-reduction techniques, as explained in the section on nicotine.

☑ Acupuncture has been used very successfully to relieve withdrawal symptoms and to assist in detoxification of heavy drugs. When acupuncture works, it creates almost immediately a sense of peace and relaxation without cravings. For programs or acupuncturists experienced in heroin detoxification, check the yellow pages of your phone book or contact the National Acupuncture Detoxification Association, 3115 Broadway, Apartment 51, New York, N.Y. 10027, 212-993-3100.

NICOTINE

From childhood you have seen ads linking cigarette smoking with a hip, young, and active lifestyle. Those gorgeous models on the billboards look so self-confident and poised with that narrow cigarette in their hands. Of course, you cannot smell their breath. And they never tell you about the problems they have caused themselves and their babies because of their habit.

Heavy smokers are half as fertile and light smokers three-quarters as fertile as the average woman, with smokers over three times more likely than nonsmokers to need more than one year to conceive. In addition, medical research has connected smoking to a 30 percent greater risk of miscarriage and twice the risk of pregnancy occurring in the fallopian tube (ectopic pregnancy) instead of the uterus. Ectopic pregnancy is a leading cause of maternal death.

Carbon monoxide in cigarettes reduces the amount of oxygen in your blood. Meanwhile, the nicotine in cigarettes constricts both your own and your baby's blood vessels, limiting even further the amount of oxygen reaching both of you. This is the reason smokers' babies tend to be small for their age.

Smoking also increases the risk of abnormal placement of the placenta in the uterus (placenta previa) and the smoker is more likely to experience heavy bleeding late in pregnancy. The more you smoke, the more abnormal your placenta will become. There is also greater risk of premature rupture of the membranes and premature birth. A smoker is more likely to need hospitalization, transfusions, and cesarean delivery.

Fathers are not exempt. Research suggests an association between a father's (as well as a mother's) smoking after birth with Sudden Infant Death Syndrome. Smoking also causes abnormal sperm in the smoker himself.

Smoking is a give-and-take experience. It gives you several thousand chemicals, some known to be carcinogenic, which have been used in the growing, curing, and preparing of the tobacco. It takes from you certain nutrients, because cigarettes reduce vitamin C, folic acid, thiamin (B-1), and calcium in the smoker's body and alter the way vitamin B-6 is used.

· W H A T   T O   D O ·

☑ Stop smoking now. Women who stop during pregnancy are more likely to avoid premature delivery and to deliver a baby of normal weight than women who continue to smoke.

☑ Stopping will be easier if you realize that smoking gives you some kind of payoff, such as reduction of stress, boredom, or hunger. Otherwise you would not smoke. You must identify that payoff, so you can arrange to receive it from a different source.

☑ Acupuncture can help eliminate cravings during that first difficult week after quitting. Not all acupuncturists, however, have learned how to treat addictions. Go only to an acupuncturist with a good track record for helping people stop smoking. Ask to speak to other patients the acupuncturist has treated.

☑ Certain herbs can help eliminate withdrawal symptoms. Try oat straw (Avena sativa), an herb that reduces symptoms of nicotine withdrawal. You can probably find an oat straw tincture in most well-stocked health-food stores.

☑ If you smoke only when under stress, relax! You can learn to handle stress differently with yoga, meditation, or biofeedback (training in reducing stress by relaxing muscles and voluntarily increasing blood flow). The benefit of meditation or biofeedback compared to vigorous exercise (which also can help) is that you can instantly achieve mental relaxation anywhere, anytime. For yoga, meditation, or biofeedback training, look in the yellow pages of your phone book or obtain videotapes and books about these techniques at local bookstores.

☑ If you have been a long-term smoker, invest in strong prenatal vitamin and mineral supplements. Catch up nutritionally by improving your daily diet.

☑ Do not drink coffee when trying to quit smoking. Smokers metabolize caffeine more quickly than nonsmokers. If you continue to drink coffee while quitting, you will have unexpected jitters since your normal two cups of coffee a day can feel like five.

☑ An excellent sourcebook for you and for your loved ones is *The No-Nag, No-Guilt, Do It Your Own Way Guide to Quitting Smoking,* by Tom Ferguson, M.D. (Random House 1989); it includes an appendix titled "How to Help a Health-Concerned Smoker." Order it from your local bookstore.

☑ Don't get discouraged. The typical successful nonsmoker quit three times before stopping permanently.

Environmental Toxicants

I t is easy to feel overwhelmed and discouraged when everything in the environment seems to be dangerous to the developing fetus. Although our air, water, and food supply do need to be monitored, it is also true that simple changes in your daily life can help to protect you and your child.

Not all the problems cited in this chapter will apply to you, and not everyone exposed to a potential danger will be adversely affected. As with every other section of this guidebook, begin with those changes that your family will find easiest to make and keep.

AIR

Outdoor Air

Pregnant women may not realize that outdoor air can be dangerous to them. For example, carbon monoxide is a tasteless, odorless, colorless gas and is one of the most significant outdoor air pollutants. Wherever you find car engines, leaf blowers, or any other combustion engine, you will find increased levels of carbon monoxide nearby. The burning of wood, coal, or natural gas also produces carbon monoxide.

When a pregnant woman breathes heavy doses of carbon monoxide, her red blood cells load up on the poison; she and her fetus receive less oxygen than they need for proper brain function.

Carbon monoxide poisoning may also contribute to babies who are small for their gestational age because women living at high altitudes (where there is less oxygen year-round) give birth to smaller-weight babies. The carbon monoxide in cigarette smoke may be to blame for the low birth weight that results from smoking during pregnancy.

Additionally, outdoor air may contain lead, which has been linked to spontaneous abortions, infertility, premature delivery, stillbirth, malformations, and serious damage to the blood and brains of fetuses. Lead exposure in the air has decreased significantly since Americans switched to unleaded gasoline, but it still exists—especially around gasoline stations and along congested highways.

Outdoor air may also contain other heavy metals, chemicals, radioactivity, and particulate matter from manufacturing plants or hazardous-waste incinerators that may affect the health of your fetus.

· W H A T   T O   D O ·

☑ Short of moving to an unpolluted area, you can protect yourself by not inhaling chemical vapors or lead dust whenever possible. See What To Do in Occupational Hazards for Women and Your Child's Environment for suggestions on how to avoid these toxicants. To prevent unnecessary exposure to carbon monoxide in your car or home, do not warm up the car engine in a garage attached to the house.

☑ If you can, avoid bumper-to-bumper traffic and congested indoor parking lots. If you cannot avoid daily rush hour traffic, you might want to invest in a car air filter or a simple fan to improve ventilation.

Indoor Air

We like to think of our homes as safe havens in a dangerous world. When the EPA sampled indoor and outdoor air from households in the West, Northeast, South, and Midwest, however, it found that some households had chemical exposures seventy times the outdoor rates. The worst dangers included cigarette smoke, air fresheners, moth crystals, aerosol sprays, paints, and solvents.

One common reason for indoor pollution is the energy-saving efforts we have all taken to weatherproof older homes and offices or to build new ones that allow little circulation between indoor and outdoor air. Furnishings, cleaning solutions, pesticides, and building materials often contain volatile organic compounds that release toxic fumes and accumulate indoors. Even low concentrations of indoor air pollution can have a cumulative effect on your pregnancy, especially considering you spend from 90 to 95 percent of your time indoors at work or at home.

Paint fumes can also be dangerous, particularly if they contain mercury, a known teratogen. Although mercury at levels of 200 parts per million or more was banned in interior paint as of August 20, 1990, stock produced before the ban may still be sold.

We may never discover every teratogenic chemical in our immediate environment for these reasons: ingredients in household cleaners, plastics, paints, and synthetic building materials are considered trade secrets, and labels do not yet list the reproductive effects of chemical ingredients; moreover, although there are well over half a million chemicals in common use, only a fraction of these have been tested for reproductive effects. Even experts have difficulty figuring out what constitutes a hazard to pregnancy, and at what exposure dose. Your best defense is to assume no chemical is safe during pregnancy if that chemical is a known danger in any other way.

· W H A T   T O   D O ·

☑ Start using nontoxic, inexpensive household cleansers. Excellent guidebooks are listed in "Occupational Hazards for Women."

☑ Check out mail-order catalogs of environmentally safe products for office, home, and landscape—such as Seventh Generation, 802-655-3116, Colchester, Vt. 05446-1672; or Ecco Bella, 800-888-5320 (201-226-5799 in New Jersey), 6 Provost Square, Apartment 602, Caldwell, N.J. 07006.

☑ If you are pregnant, do not paint the nursery. Have someone else do the work using nontoxic and odor-free paints whenever possible. Keep the windows open and stay out of the house until there is no paint odor. If you use interior latex paint, it is important to ventilate your home thoroughly and to ask for proof that the paint you buy does not contain mercury.

☑ Avoid smoke-filled rooms to protect your fetus from lack of oxygen. In metropolitan areas throughout the United States, background carbon monoxide levels hover around 40 to 50 parts per million (ppm). In a fume-laden garage or tunnel, carbon monoxide may reach 100 ppm. In a room filled with cigarette smoke, levels of carbon monoxide can reach several hundred parts per million.

☑ To measure a five- to seven-day sample of air for formaldehyde levels in your home or office, obtain the PF-1 formaldehyde monitor kit (contains two monitors) from Air Quality Research, P.O. Box 14063, Research Triangle Park, N.C. 27709, 800-242-7472 ($60.50 postpaid).

☑ Have household appliances checked for gas leaks. Use a vent or open a window while cooking on a gas range. Ditto for drying clothes and heating with a kerosene space heater. Better yet, avoid using kerosene space heaters, which pollute your home with carbon monoxide, formaldehyde, sulfur dioxide, and other chemical vapors. One EPA official calls them outrageous dangers for pregnant women.

☑ A variety of houseplants help with pollution control by absorbing and transforming pollutants—such as formaldehyde, carbon monoxide, benzene, carbon dioxide, cigarette smoke, and other airborne toxicants—through their leaves and roots with the help of microorganisms in the soil. If you can handle only one plant, make it a chrysanthemum, according to William Wolverton, Ph.D., an environmental scientist who did the original research on plant filtration.

☑ If you would rather purchase an electric air filter, be aware that different systems absorb different pollutants. Before investing in an expensive filter, read Debra Lynn Dadd's *Nontoxic, Natural, & Earthwise* (Tarcher 1991) for an excellent discussion of products and suppliers.

☑ Other guidebooks that can help include the following:
   House Dangerous: Indoor Pollution in Your Home and Office and What You Can Do About It!, by Ellen J. Greenfield (Vintage 1987). An excellent sourcebook on pollutants, legal liability, recipes for natural alternatives, and how to easily reduce toxins in your home.
   The Healthy House: How to Buy One, How to Cure a Sick One, How to Build One, by John Bower (Lyle Stuart 1989). Good for those who want to start from scratch.
   Guide to Hazardous Products Around the Home: A Personal Action Manual for Protecting Your Health and Environment,

published by Household Hazardous Waste Project (1989): HHWP, 1031 East Battlefield, Apartment 214, Springfield, MO 65807 ($9.95 postpaid). Describes how to recognize, eliminate, and find alternatives to everyday hazardous waste. Excellent resources section.

Chemical Exposures, by Nicholas A. Ashford and Claudia S. Miller (Van Nostrand Reinhold, 1990), based on a landmark study by the New Jersey Department of Health on the subject of chemical exposures and public health. The price is $18.95.

WATER

Not all tap water is contaminated, but according to the Center for Science in the Public Interest, in 1988 more than 11 million Americans drank tap water containing illegal levels of contaminants. Some of those contaminants endanger the fetus and newborn. Happily, we can find out for ourselves how clean our water is and, if necessary, improve its quality.

Lead and Other Metals

A study conducted by the EPA in 1986 revealed up to 40 percent of the lead threatening the health of Americans is found in their tap water. The study concluded that as many as one out of every five Americans served by a municipal water utility had lead in their drinking water.

There is really no safe lead level. In 1984, Herbert L. Needleman, M.D., from the School of Medicine, University of Pittsburgh, reported a link between lead contamination and birth defects. Needleman and his colleagues found that malformations were more likely as the percent of lead in the infant's umbilical cord blood increased.

What is so devastating about lead is not only its potential to create malformations but also its influence on the physical and mental development of the child. In later studies, Needleman and his colleagues reported that children who were contaminated in the womb by their mothers' lead exposure had more serious developmental consequences than did children who were exposed to lead directly, during their first two years of life. Other studies clearly link lead contamination to diminished intelligence in children.

In 1991 federal standards for lead in drinking water were lowered from

50 ppm to 15 ppm and for the definition of lead poisoning in children from 25 micrograms of lead per deciliter of blood to 10 micrograms.

The most common source of lead in water is your own home plumbing. Copper pipes can contain up to 50 percent lead in their solder, but build-up of sediment over at least five years may prevent lead from leaching out at the joints. Turn-of-the-century plumbing, on the other hand, may be entirely of lead, and with so much surface area the sediment may not help.

The federal government prohibited the use of lead in pipes and solder in 1986, but states had until 1988 to begin enforcing the ban. As a result, some new homes and very old homes are at greatest risk for lead in tap water.

Mercury

Methylmercury is a known teratogen and, in 1955, was to blame for deaths, cerebral palsy, and other birth defects along Minamata Bay, in Japan. A chemical plant dumped industrial waste that contained inorganic mercury into the bay. Microorganisms converted the inorganic mercury to methylmercury. Algae took up the compound, and fish consumed the algae. Pregnant women then consumed the fish; it is a clearcut example of how environmental toxins move up the food chain. Unfortunately, methylmercury poisoning also occurred elsewhere in Japan, as well as in New Mexico and the Great Lakes region of the United States. Tuna, swordfish, and shark are known to accumulate mercury, as do eels, northern pike, striped bass, and walleye when exposed to industrial effluents. Because of high levels of methylmercury in fish, federal, state, and municipal regulations restrict sport and commercial fishing in numerous lakes and rivers in both Canada and the United States.

Chemical Contamination

Aquifers deep underground were once considered a safer source of drinking water than surface water, but during the 1980s it was found they had been contaminated by agricultural and industrial runoff. Some of the most common contaminants are DBCP (dibromochloropropane), a soil fumigant that is toxic to sperm, and three halogenated chlorine solvents: PCE (perchloroethylene), which is used by dry cleaners, TCA (1.1.1-trichloroethane), and TCE (trichloroethylene). Birth defects have been reported when pregnant women consumed water contaminated with these chemicals in Woburn, Massachusetts; Tucson, Arizona; Gray, Maine; and a number of other U.S. cities.

While investigating a reported chemical leak in Santa Clara County,

California, the California Department of Health Services discovered that women who drank bottled or filtered water instead of city tap water during pregnancy had a significantly lower rate of spontaneous abortion and birth defects. A follow-up study undertaken with Kaiser-Permanente Division of Research revealed that the risk of miscarriage was 50 percent greater among those who drink tap water compared to those who do not. In applying this county's experience to your own, you will need to compare the quality of water offered by local bottlers to that supplied by your municipality.

Radiation

Radon is a radioactive gas that seeps into water systems from deep within the earth. "I worry more about it [radon] than about all the other potential carcinogens in drinking water combined," says Bruce Macler, Ph.D., an EPA toxicologist specializing in water contamination.

Radium, another radioactive substance that originates in certain rocks, is also found in drinking water in the United States, though to a lesser extent than radon. Where it does exist, it can cause birth defects and cancer. For example, Lois Haertel and Linda Baer, from South Dakota State University, estimated that about 30 percent of childhood cancer in South Dakota was due to naturally occurring radiation in tap water, and that these cases might be avoided by simply removing the toxic substances from the children's water supply. Recent studies performed in North Carolina linked radium in drinking water to growing rates of childhood leukemia in that state. And in New York State, where a connection between radium in drinking water and birth defects was discovered thirty-four years ago, the rate of birth defects dropped to nearly normal in areas where residents drank water from streams and lakes rather than from wells and springs, which had more likelihood of radiation contamination.

· W H A T   T O   D O ·

☑ Get your water tested. Not all tap water is polluted enough to warrant your spending money on an alternative. The cost of tests varies from less than fifty dollars to several hundred dollars. Probably the most dangerous water sources are private wells, which can be contaminated by septic systems, animal wastes, agricultural chemicals, and radon.

Look in your local phone book under Laboratories-testing for sources of water tests, or contact one of the following companies, which specialize in water testing and therefore may offer you a more competitive price: National Testing Laboratories, Cleveland, Ohio, 800-458-3330; Suburban Water Testing Laboratories, Temple, Pa., 800-433-6595; and WaterTest Corporation of Manchester, N.H., 800-H2O-TEST (425-8378).

☑ Ask the public relations department of your local water utility for a printed form comparing its laboratory findings to the federal safety standard. For a brochure titled *Is Your Drinking Water Safe?*, which lists the federal standards for drinking water contaminants, and one titled *Lead in Your Drinking Water*, call the EPA Safe Drinking Water Hotline at 800-426-4791.

☑ Ask local bottled-water companies for their water's analysis and compare companies to one another and to your city's tap water. Tap water is regulated by the National Interim Primary Drinking Water Regulations of 1975, but bottled water isn't regulated by federal standards unless the water is sold across state lines. So don't assume bottled water is of higher quality until you see the proof.

☑ Test your water before purchasing a water filter. You must know what needs to be removed so you'll know what type of filter to buy. An activated carbon block filter will remove pesticides, chlorine, trihalomethanes, industrial solvents, and radon gas but you need a reverse osmosis unit to remove nitrates or lead. For excellent advice see either *Nontoxic, Natural, & Earthwise* by Debra Lynn Dadd (Tarcher 1990), or *Diet for a Poisoned Planet* by David Steinman (Harmony 1990).

☑ If lead is your water's major problem and your own pipes are your home's source of lead, replace the pipes. (It may be the responsibility of your local utility to do so.)

☑ Scientists in the U.S., Canada, and Japan have discovered natural detoxifiers which you can easily add to your daily meals. Garlic and onions help remove both lead and mercury. Seaweeds (including kelp tablets) bind to lead in the intestines and help remove it. Eating foods rich in calcium, iron, and zinc helps reduce absorption of lead, and reduces symptoms of lead toxicity. Food sources of these minerals include: seafoods (especially oysters and herring), lean meat, yogurt, egg yolks, pumpkin and sunflower seeds, brazil nuts, garbanzo beans, blackeyed peas, and wheat germ.

☑ Get yourself and your children screened for levels of lead in your blood if your home was built before 1978.

☑ During pregnancy, you may want to limit your consumption of fish known to be mercury-accumulators, such as shark, swordfish, tuna, northern pike, walleye, eels, and striped bass unless you are sure they originated in unpolluted waters.

HIDDEN CONTAMINATION

Lead: Besides water and outdoor air, common household sources of lead contamination include dust, dolomite, colored newspaper print, metallic wrapping paper inks, print on bread bags, leaded ceramic glazes (especially on foreign-bought pottery), and crystal glassware.

Mercury: Around 100 million Americans have silver fillings (amalgam), which are 50 percent inorganic mercury, in their mouths. This is a different form than the organic methylmercury that accumulates in fish, yet it is still toxic to the environment. The Environmental Protection Agency and local authorities have initiated court action against dentists who improperly disposed of scrap amalgam.

Minute amounts of mercury in vapor or particulate form can release from silver-mercury amalgam fillings when you eat acidic foods or gnash your teeth. The American Dental Association maintains that because this source of the heavy metal is minuscule it is not dangerous. A report by the World Health Organization, however, suggests that women of childbearing age should reduce their exposure to mercury vapor as much as possible as there is no good research proving the material is safe. Meanwhile, an official health agency in Sweden has identified amalgam as "toxic and unsuitable as a dental filling material" and has recommended that "to prevent mercury damage to the fetus" pregnant women should not be given amalgam restorations. It appears that some percent of the population is especially sensitive to the metal.

Landfills or dumps: Love Canal opened our eyes to the potential danger of living on or near waste dumps, even when those dumps have been filled, covered, and used for public institutions. The Love Canal tract, near Niagara Falls, New York, was used as a dump by a chemical company, then sold to the city as a landfill. Over the next twenty-five years, about 250 different chemicals seeped into basements, schoolyards, and sewers that were built on the site. Some residents believed that their health problems, including birth defects, miscarriages, babies with low birth weight, and childhood cancers were the result of their contaminated neighborhood. A communitywide organization was formed and gained national attention. As a result, Congress created the 1980 Superfund law providing money to clean up dangerously contaminated sites.

· W H A T   T O   D O ·

☑ Obtain an inexpensive kit to do a test for lead in your home. One company whose kits are known to be reliable is Lead-Check, P.O. Box 1210, Framingham, Mass. 01701, 800-262-LEAD. Ask if their test for lead in water is on the market yet.

   The most reliable test for lead uses an X-ray Fluorescence (XRF) Spectrum Analyzer. XRF is recommended by the U.S. Department of Housing and Urban Development (HUD). Your local health department may provide this service or refer you to an appropriate professional for the test.

☑ Do not eat or drink from pottery bought abroad until it is tested for lead. Never drink from crystal. (In 1991 two professors at Columbia University found that lead levels doubled in white wine held in a lead-crystal goblet for only one hour. Crystal will release lead into other beverages, too.)

☑ Use trisodium phosphate (TSP) detergent on floors and window sills frequently and pick up excess water with a wet/dry shop-model vacuum cleaner.

☑ It is difficult to clean all of the collected lead dust from carpets. Your best choice is a hardwood floor and modestly priced washable cotton rugs.

☑ For information on the safety of dental amalgam, contact the American Dental Association, 211 East Chicago, Chicago, Ill. 60611, 800-621-8099. For information on amalgam's dangers, obtain a copy of a television segment from *60 Minutes* on the subject titled "Is There Poison in Your Mouth?" It aired December 6, 1990, and is available from Ambrose Video Publishing, 800-843-0048. Contact either the Toxic Element Research Foundation in Colorado Springs, Colo. (800-331-2303) for *It's All in Your Head: Diseases Caused by Silver-Mercury Fillings,* by Hal A. Huggins, D.D.S. ($10); or the Environmental Dental Association in San Diego, Calif. (800-388-8124) for *The Complete Guide to Mercury Toxicity from Dental Fillings: How to Find Out If Your Silver Dental Fillings Are Poisoning You and What You Can Do about It,* by Joyal Taylor, D.D.S. ($15). Both organizations will help you find out who in your area can discuss the pros and cons of dental amalgams with you.

☑ To find out if there is a toxic dump beneath your home or anywhere else, San Franciscan Janice England, of People Investigating Toxic Sites (PITS), suggests first inspecting the property for discolored soil or abnormal growth of foliage, then searching government agencies for maps of dump sites, the names and businesses of previous owners, reports on chemical testing done on the soil, and building permits that describe any fill under the property at the time of construction.

Also helpful is the nonprofit Citizen's Clearinghouse for Hazardous Wastes, which provides information and training to individuals and neighborhood groups concerned about toxic-waste issues: CCHW, P.O. Box 6806, Falls Church, Va. 22040, 703-237-2249.

ELECTROMAGNETIC RADIATION

It is easier to discuss the risk of birth defects caused by electromagnetism if we divide the radiation spectrum into two parts: ionizing and nonionizing.

Ionizing Radiation

Ionizing radiation is composed of short waves of energy that vibrate at very high frequencies. These rays can reach us through radioactive radon and radium (in some water, indoor air, or building materials), cosmic rays (especially in mountain communities or during air travel), nuclear weapons fallout, and medical X rays.

As with every other environmental hazard, if a woman receives ionizing radiation from any source during the first two weeks after conception, the embryo may repair itself and develop normally. If irradiated during the critical nine weeks when organs are developing, intrauterine growth retardation, mental retardation, cancer, and skeletal and central nervous system abnormalities may result—depending on the dose, the nutritional status of the woman and fetus, and other factors.

To understand why this occurs, recall from high-school science that the definition of an ion is *a charged particle* and that an atom's electric charge is neutral because its positively charged nucleus is perfectly balanced by the appropriate number of negatively charged electrons whizzing around it. When ionizing radiation passes through atoms of living tissue, the radiation jerks electrons out of their orbits, changing the formerly neutral atom to a positive charge—ionizing it. The freed electrons are expelled with such force that they rip other electrons off other atoms in a cascade of destruction. At some level there is damage to chromosomes, the structures in the nucleus of every cell that contain DNA, our genetic blueprint. In many cases, the DNA can repair itself before the damage becomes permanent. Trouble arises from injuries that are irreparable or improperly repaired in the DNA of a fetus.

In 1986 British researchers George W. Kneale and Alice M. Stewart, of Birmingham, England, concluded that prenatal exposure to background ionizing radiation was the single most important cause of juvenile cancer in England, accounting for at least 75 percent of childhood cancers, especially leukemia. The two sources of radiation exposure that will most concern American parents are those in the home and in medical offices. Specifically, Kneale and Stewart found that 15 to 20 percent of all juvenile cancers were due to terrestrial sources of radiation, which includes uranium breakdown products such as radon and radium in the water supply and radon from other sources, and 6 to 7 percent were due to medical X rays during pregnancy. Where fetal exposure was high and yet cancer did not develop, they found it common for children to die from infectious diseases, instead, which the authors suggest was due to radiation's effect on the children's immune system.

This does not mean that radiation should be avoided at all cost. Radiation can guide medical care to save your life and to reduce complications of disease or injury. Nevertheless, it is a tool to be used judiciously. It is not farfetched to imagine someone living in a home polluted with radon gas, whose drinking water contains radon or radium, who inhales radioactive lead-210 and polonium-210 in every cigarette puff, who receives diagnostic X rays after a car accident and is exposed to continuous albeit minute doses of ionizing radiation in a variety of hidden ways, including thorium in eyeglass lenses and cerium-laced porcelain dental crowns (with an approximate yearly local dose of 1 rem a year per crown).

Erik Jansson, director of the National Network to Prevent Birth Defects, figures that by halving the American average exposure to ionizing radiation, the United States can save around 3.3 billion dollars a year in costs of genetic disease and birth defects and 1 billion dollars a year in costs of mental retardation and learning disabilities.

· W H A T   T O   D O ·

☑ Limit your exposure to sources of radiation. The National Council on Radiation Protection (NCRP) recommends that women who work with or around radiation limit their exposure for the entire pregnancy to no more than 0.5 rem. For comparison, one dental side view X ray delivers 0.513 rems, and one abdominal X ray delivers 0.6 rems.

☑ Avoid needless X rays. Obtain a second opinion before undergoing any non-emergency X rays during pregnancy or labor. Any time you are X rayed, insist upon shielding your ovaries (and for men, testicles) with a lead apron. Obtain a copy of *X rays: Health Effects of Common Exams,* by John W. Gofman, M.D., Ph.D., and Egan O'Connor (Sierra Club Books 1985). This very practical reference offers you a clear explanation of the potential risk of many different dental and medical exams for various ages, from fetus to adult.

☑ Laboratory testing is the only way to verify radioactive elements in tap water. Companies that test water are listed under the section "Water." Radon as a gas is measurable using test kits obtained through hardware stores or referrals from your local health department or lung association.

☑ If the air in your home measures above 4 pCi/1 of radon gas with a simple home-test kit, you may want to call the EPA for a list of companies that have passed the EPA Radon Measurement Proficiency Program. If their more sophisticated tests confirm your cheaper one, it is time to stop radon from entering the foundation of your house.

You can also obtain from the EPA a list of companies that have passed the EPA Radon Contractor Proficiency Program, or, if you want to do the work yourself, you can obtain free EPA booklets on the subject. Call the EPA Radon Hotline at 800-767-7236.

☑ Seaweeds not only help eliminate lead from the body but, according to research published in the *Canadian Medical Association Journal,* seaweeds such as kelp and kombu also help protect you from the effects of ionizing radiation. So, add them to your soup to maximize your body's nutritional defense.

☑ Read *Everybody's Radiation Handbook,* by Steve M. Dean (Aeon Research Co. 1989). Available from ARC, 114 Nicholl Avenue, Point Richmond, Calif. 94801 ($6.95 postpaid).

Nonionizing Radiation

Nonionizing radiation refers to the energy coming out of wall sockets, radio and television transmission towers, and microwave dishes. It is nonionizing because it is so weak it cannot knock electrons off atomic nuclei. Even a weak current of electricity, however, creates both an electric field and a magnetic field around the current, collectively called an electromagnetic field.

Whether or not a nonionizing electromagnetic field is harmful to pregnant women and others is still highly controversial. For a century, scientists have assumed that the only danger of nonionizing electromagnetic energy was heat. We have harnessed that heat in microwave ovens, peppered our landscape with transmission towers, and cluttered our lives with electronic devices for every conceivable convenience. Thirty years of research on animals and epidemiological studies of human populations, however, are leading some scientists to conclude that chronic, albeit minute, exposure to electromagnetic energy fields might influence reproduction, contribute to childhood and adult cancer, and damage our health in other ways.

Pioneering research by Dr. Nancy Wertheimer, of the University of Colorado Medical Center, suggests that pregnant women chronically exposed to magnetic fields created by electric blankets or ceiling-cable electric heating units have a greater likelihood of miscarriage.

Studies of the possible harm to pregnant women of radiation emitted by video display terminals (VDTs) have been utterly confusing, with most disproving any connection between VDT work and miscarriage but some suggesting there may be a link. In one large study published in the *New England Journal of Medicine* in 1991, women in the control group who did not use VDTs were exposed to the same extremely low-frequency (ELF) electromagnetic fields as those who used VDTs. So although the use of VDTs themselves did not appear to increase the rate of miscarriage, the study still did not answer the question whether ELF fields cause miscarriage. A study in progress at Mt. Sinai School of Medicine will provide more information on the effect of ELFs on miscarriage and fertility, but results will not be available for some time.

Research to date suggests that magnetic fields may be more worrisome than electric fields. Unlike toxic chemicals—where if a little is bad, more is worse—electromagnetic radiation seems to have specific doses at which effects appear and then disappear as power is increased. There are many questions still to be answered before power companies and government agencies know the best actions to take. Meanwhile, since research suggests electromagnetic radiation may not be harmless, the most conservative approach is to pursue what electric power utilities call prudent avoidance.

· W H A T   T O   D O ·

☑ Eliminate unnecessary exposure. Prudent avoidance means reducing your exposure to both electric and magnetic fields without spending a lot of money. Unplug unused appliances. Use your hair dryer only when really necessary and at other times let your hair dry naturally. When you do use an electric dryer, use lower settings (magnetic fields are higher at higher settings) and hold the hair dryer as far away as practical from your body. Use several blankets instead of one electric blanket or heat the bed, then unplug the blanket before going to sleep. Insulate your waterbed with layered blankets and a thick mattress cover instead of using an electric heater. Move beds to indoor walls that are not opposite outside electrical circuit boxes.

☑ Reduce necessary exposure. Since field strengths fall rather rapidly with distance from their source, keep a good six feet from your television set and at least an arm's length away from any side of a computer monitor. Non–back-lit LCD (liquid-crystal display) screens (often used in laptop computers) do not use a cathode ray tube and therefore do not create a magnetic field. The laptop may be a viable alternative if you or your company are planning to acquire new monitors soon. Or, when purchasing a new full-size monitor, look for one that meets Swedish emission standards (which are higher than American standards). If you do not need a color monitor, use a black-and-white model, since these generally give off less radiation. Also, shut off unused monitors. For further advice, call the 9 to 5 National Association of Working Women hotline: 800-245-9865 10 A.M. to 4 P.M. EST. Ask for their four-page handout on VDTs, Pregnancy, and Radiation. Or, write 9 to 5, 614 Superior Avenue N.W., Cleveland, Ohio 44113. If you're a photo editor who stares at slides through a photo loupe, be aware that being an inch or two from a lightbox can expose you to the same intensity of magnetic field experienced by electricians, power line workers, and welders. Reduce your exposure by having an electrician remove the ballast and put it at the end of a cord extending several feet away. Or, bring the transparency up to the loupe at your eye. Two feet from the lightbox the field strength is less than 2 mG.

☑ In the studies linking magnetic fields to a higher risk of childhood leukemia, constant exposure to 2.5 to 3 milligauss (mG) was generally found to be the danger threshold. Borrow a gaussmeter from your local power utility and measure handheld and major home appliances, the head and center of your bed, various walls, and so on to get an idea of the variety of magnetic field strengths to which you are regularly exposed. Remember, take readings in several directions at each site, as electromagnetic fields are three dimensional.

☑ If you are buying a new home, one factor among others to consider is its proximity to high-power transmission lines. For pro on the issue, contact your local power company. For con, read *Cross Currents*, by Robert O. Becker, M.D. (Tarcher 1990), and *Currents of Death*, by Paul Brodeur (Simon & Schuster 1989).

PESTICIDES

Pesticide contamination is potentially dangerous for the pregnant woman. These poisons are found in small quantities in our food supply; moreover, we frequently spray them indoors and around the yard without a thought to their effects. In fact, more than 90 percent of households in the United States use pesticides. Perhaps fewer people would use them if they knew household pesticides have been linked to increased risk of childhood leukemia, brain cancer, neuroblastoma (a cancerous tumor), and malformed limbs.

When considering the potential danger of any chemical, it is necessary to distinguish between acute toxic doses and chronic lower-level exposure. There is no question that direct exposure to pesticides is an obvious cause of birth defects and cancer, but chronic exposure can also lead to cancer, genetic changes, or even birth defects. For example, deformed limbs among children of agricultural workers in California were found thirteen times more frequently than among the general population.

Pesticides are not flushed out of the body. They remain inside human cells, accumulating in the brain, bones, liver, intestines, fat, and lymphatics. People vary in their susceptibility to pesticide poisoning depending on their genetic makeup, nutrition, immune system, and other toxins to which they are simultaneously exposed.

In addition to active ingredients, each pesticide contains varying quantities of chemicals considered inert because they do not kill pests. So-called inert chemicals include well-known carcinogens, such as benzene, asbestos, and carbon tetrachloride, plus suspected carcinogens, such as formaldehyde. Since the inert chemicals are considered trade secrets, you will not find them listed on the label.

Unfortunately, pesticides considered "legal" were inadequately tested for behavioral and neurological effects. According to a 1984 report from the National Academy of Sciences, 90 percent of all pesticides sold in America have not been adequately tested for damage to the nervous system; 71 to 80 percent have not been adequately tested for cancer; 51 to 60 percent have not been adequately tested for birth defects; and 21 to 30 percent have not been adequately tested for genetic mutations.

· W H A T   T O   D O ·

☑ Avoid direct exposure to any pesticide. Do not use them around the house or garden unless you have a serious problem with pests. If you do use pesticides, keep food, kitchen supplies, children, and pets away from sprayed areas and do not inhale the spray yourself. Alternatively, use natural pesticides. Try spraying your plants with a mixture of two ounces Ivory soap to one gallon water. There are several fine catalogs selling nontoxic alternatives to pesticides, including Gardens Alive!, Highway 48, P.O. Box 149, Sunman, Ind. 47041, 812-623-4201.

☑ Buy in-season produce grown close to home or certified organic produce. There is no standard definition of organic food. We generally assume it means raised without pesticides, but what one state defines as organic does not necessarily conform to stricter standards in another state. You can feel most assured if the produce has been certified by an independent organization or state agency.

☑ Wash chemical residues off of fruits and vegetables and avoid produce from tropical countries, because they are prone to mold and fungi and therefore are more often treated with fungicides. Foreign countries, in addition, often use pesticides that are banned in the United States.

☑ For the known effect of specific pesticides on the environment and health, call the National Pesticide Telecommunications Network at 800-858-7378. Information is available twenty-four hours a day, seven days a week.

☑ Educate yourself on the issue. Read *Pesticide Alert,* by Lawrie Mott and Karen Snyder (Sierra Club Books 1987), which lists commonly used pesticides known to produce reproductive toxicity and birth defects. Also see *Diet for a Poisoned Planet,* by David Steinman (Harmony 1990), or *Safe Food,* by Michael P. Jacobson, Ph.D., Lisa Y. Lefferts, and Anne Witte Garland (Center for Science in the Public Interest 1991), available in bookstores.

Exercise

Once upon a time pregnant women were urged to avoid strenuous activity, including exercise. There was fear of causing a miscarriage or
even deformities due to jarring movements, the shunting of oxygen-rich
blood away from the uterus and into muscles of the woman's arms and legs,
and increased body heat. But today scientific experimentation has proven
these fears groundless, and pregnant women are no longer urged to take it
easy. Although an expanding belly does slow them down, pregnant
women receive important benefits from regular exercise.

Before pregnancy, an active woman enjoys cardiovascular fitness,
lowered tension, and an attractive body. During pregnancy, she experiences minimal problems with varicose veins, leg cramps, sleepless nights,
sore back, and constipation. She may also have more energy, be more in
tune with her body, and feel more confident of its physical abilities than
does the inactive woman. Although not all studies suggest women who are
physically fit have shorter, less complicated labors, there is no indication
that even vigorous exercise harms the fetus, as long as the mother is pursu-
ing activities of the same general intensity as she did before pregnancy.

The experience of women who take to the roads, pools, and dance
floors during pregnancy has been to some degree confirmed by the studies
of James F. Clapp, III, M.D., an obstetrician and researcher at Metro-
Health Medical Center in Cleveland, Ohio. Clapp found no increased risk
of miscarriage, placental problems, prematurity, or structural abnormalities in the children of runners and aerobic dancers who had been exercising for at least two years before becoming pregnant and who averaged
from one and a half to six hours a week of vigorous exercise during pregnancy.

Some studies have found slightly lower birth weight among babies of
women who exercised strenuously during their entire pregnancy. Clapp

found that baby size was related to the intensity and amount of exercise during the pregnancy, compared to the woman's prepregnancy level. If an athlete does not cut down her time and distance during the second half of her pregnancy, her baby will be smaller, by about a pound and a half, than if she does reduce her exercise program.

It is important to note that the reports on exercise are relative to the individual. "For example," explains Clapp, "if you take a lady running 60 miles a week before she's pregnant who cuts back to 30 miles a week during pregnancy, she's going to have a big baby. If a lady runs 20 miles a week before pregnancy and continues to run 20 miles a week during pregnancy, her baby will be smaller than it would have been had she cut back."

Weight is not the only concern. What about brain size? The brains of the athletes' newborns were just as big, as measured by head circumference, as those of nonathletes. The babies were also as long; they were just leaner.

What actually happens to the fetus while the mother is exercising? His normal heart rate of 120 to 160 beats per minute rises 10 to 20 beats a minute, depending on how hard the mother is working and how long she works. The baby moves more in the womb, which helps him develop his muscles and nerves. When the pregnant woman's endorphins kick in, meaning those great neurochemicals that create feelings of peace and euphoria, some percentage passes through the placenta and enters the baby's circulatory system, as well. Baby gets a runners high along with Mom.

The women in Clapp's study population were already fit when they began pregnancy. His results may not universally hold true in all types of activities or among unfit women who suddenly decide to become fit now that they are pregnant. Nevertheless, his research suggests that exercise is more than simply not harmful—it is downright beneficial to the development of the unborn child. It seems possible that exercise during early pregnancy stimulates the growth of the placenta; it also appears that the woman's physiological response to heat changes, making it easier for her to get rid of heat generated by exercise than it was before she was pregnant.

Think of it this way: If vigorous exercise, including bouncing and jarring movements as in skiing, diving, and running, could easily cause abortion, a lot of unwanted children would not have been born. Over the centuries, women have tried all manner of ways to abort and have found how very securely the fetus is cushioned in its bag of waters. This is not true in cases of threatened miscarriage or premature labor, but in most cases, the baby is in there for the duration; your activity during pregnancy will only enhance the health of you both. So stop worrying and keep moving.

· W H A T   T O   D O ·

☑ Exercise is a good idea for most pregnant women. Almost everyone can at least walk, swim, do yoga, or cycle on a stationary bicycle. If you have any of the following conditions, however, you are safest getting your physician's approval before beginning any form of exercise: a history of miscarriages, premature delivery, or surgery on your uterus; obstetrical complications, such as vaginal bleeding or incompetent cervix; carrying more than one fetus; uterine contractions or ruptured membranes; or hypertension, any other heart or cardiovascular problem, diabetes, thyroid disease, or anemia.

☑ Do not exercise flat on your back during the second and third trimesters. The weight of your abdomen can compress and interfere with blood flow through a major blood vessel—the inferior vena cava—which carries blood up to your heart. This, in turn, might reduce the blood pumped to the placenta.

☑ When you ask for others' advice about exercise during pregnancy, realize that their advice may be based on personal bias. You will feel much more self-confident about your exercise program if you have read supportive scientific information, including personal experiences of pregnant exercisers found in *Woman-Centered Pregnancy and Birth*, by Ginny Cassidy-Brinn, R.N., Francie Hornstein, and Carol Downer (Cleis Press 1984).

☑ During aerobic workouts, check if you can exercise and still carry on a conversation, even if a bit breathlessly. If you can, you are not overdoing it. If you cannot talk and exercise at the pace you have set, cut back until you can.

☑ There are three useful exercise videotapes specifically for the pregnant woman:
"The American College of Obstetricians and Gynecologists Pregnancy Exercise Program," produced by Art Ulene, M.D. (51 minutes). Exercise only.

"Kathy Smith's Pregnancy Workout" (Media Home Entertainment, 90 minutes). Exercise, motivation, posture, and information on pregnancy and recovery.

"Jane Fonda's New Pregnancy Workout" (Lorimar, 50 minutes). Exercise, labor tips, and baby massage.

Gestational Diabetes

Pregnancy-induced diabetes, called gestational diabetes, occurs in about 50 out of 1000 pregnancies. You can usually control it by changing your eating habits, but some women may also need insulin injections. Because gestational diabetes usually develops in middle or late pregnancy after the fetus's organs have developed, structural birth defects seldom result. Respiratory and other problems in the fetus can result, however, as well as damage of the pregnant woman's eyes, kidneys, and cardiovascular system, so it is important to diagnose and treat gestational diabetes properly. Fortunately, the condition usually disappears at delivery.

Diabetes is a disease of abnormally high blood sugar. Our body breaks down food in the intestines into a simple form of sugar called glucose, which moves from the intestinal tract into the bloodstream. Glucose then passes from the bloodstream into every cell of the body, where it is either used by the cells as an immediate source of energy or stored in the muscles and liver for future use.

The only way glucose can pass through a cell membrane into a cell is with the help of the hormone insulin, which also helps the liver store the glucose as glycogen. Insulin is produced by specialized areas on the surface of the pancreas called beta cells.

In diabetes, the beta cells may not secrete enough insulin. Extra glucose builds up in your bloodstream and you have symptoms of high blood sugar (hyperglycemia), such as excessive urination and thirst. Severe cases may lead to coma. Sometimes, too much insulin is secreted, and so too much glucose is pulled out of the blood. In this case, you experience low blood sugar (hypoglycemia), with such symptoms as confusion, sweating, anxiety, quickened heartbeat, even convulsions and coma.

Why do some women suddenly develop this condition during pregnancy? Control of glucose slips somewhat during every pregnancy. Most women's insulin levels remain within normal range, but sometimes there is an inherited tendency toward insulin deficiency. This condition may only express itself when insulin production is challenged by the demands of the growing fetus. Physiological stresses inherent in pregnancy may affect insulin secretion; hormones can interfere with it, as can other factors that are unique to a woman's biochemistry and life situation.

Women with an increased risk of developing gestational diabetes include those who have experienced one of the following conditions:

- gestational diabetes in a prior pregnancy
- delivery of a baby larger than nine pounds
- delivery of a malformed baby
- developing excess amniotic fluid (polyhydramnios)
- unexplained stillbirth
- have grandparents, parents, children, or siblings with diabetes
- are more than 20 percent over their desirable body weight
- are age thirty-five or older

If you fall into one of these categories, you may want to ask your physician to screen you for high blood sugar early in your pregnancy.

· W H A T   T O   D O ·

☑ Watch yourself for warning signs: excessive thirst, dizziness, frequent urination.

☑ If you are diagnosed with gestational diabetes and have had no previous experience with the disease, it is especially important to stay in touch with your physician, diabetes educator, and dietician to control the condition through your diet or through insulin injections. Get your questions answered so you can manage problems early.

☑ After delivery, check your blood glucose at random times during the first few weeks to be sure your gestational diabetes has disappeared. It is also important to be tested as soon as your menstrual period starts again and when you stop breast-feeding, as hormone changes can affect test results. Since you

are more likely to develop gestational diabetes with subsequent pregnancies, alert your obstetrician to your history of
the condition at your first prenatal visit. He or she may want
to screen you earlier than usual for diabetes.

☑ Women who develop gestational diabetes and are overweight
are more likely than others to develop Type II diabetes mellitus
later in life. They should pay careful attention to diet and exercise. Remaining overweight during the years after delivery
results in a 60 percent chance of developing diabetes; staying
at an ideal weight decreases the risk to 25 percent.

Infectious Diseases

G iven that pregnant women may have other children or may often be around children, an awareness of the potential danger of infectious diseases is vital. An infectious disease contracted by the mother can be acquired by the fetus during pregnancy or during the descent through the birth canal. Not all infectious diseases can damage unborn babies, but some can. The following is a description of several common infectious diseases, a description of their possible danger, and the best ways for a mother to prevent exposure and infection while pregnant. (See "Pre-existing Medical Conditions" for a discussion of AIDS.)

CHICKEN POX (VARICELLA)

Chicken pox is practically unavoidable, as it is highly contagious and very common among schoolage children up to about age eight—though it may be contracted at any age. The disease most often occurs in winter or spring, and epidemics reappear every two to five years. Once someone catches chicken pox, he or she is usually immune for life to a recurrence of the disease.

After a chicken pox first expresses itself as a headache, fever, and tiredness. After about three days and for the next two to six days, a red rash appears anywhere on the body, but especially on the trunk. The rash develops as blisters that crust over and disappear within two weeks.

After a chicken pox infection ends, the virus apparently enters deep into nerve cells and stays there—to appear again in some people later in life as herpes zoster (shingles). Zoster expresses itself as a painful band of small, fluid-filled blisters usually along one side of the trunk or face. The Centers for Disease Control estimate that around 3.5 million cases of chicken pox and around 300,000 cases of herpes zoster occur each year in the United States.

Pregnant women who are not immune to chicken pox are at risk of severe complications, including pneumonia. The risk of birth defects are thought to be less than 1 percent when chicken pox occurs during the first half of pregnancy. In rare cases, chicken pox can produce congenital varicella syndrome in a fetus, especially during the first trimester, including severe scarring leading to malformations and growth retardation. A second time of danger is immediately after birth, when a varicella infection can even be fatal since the newborn's immune system is still immature. If the mother has contracted the disease at the very end of her pregnancy, she has not had time to develop and pass on to her fetus antibodies against the virus. According to the CDC, however, after the first couple days of life a healthy full-term baby who develops chicken pox is not known to be at any greater risk of complications than older children.

· W H A T   T O   D O ·

☑ The safest course for pregnant women who have not themselves ever had the disease is to avoid exposure to infected or recently exposed children until the children are clear of chicken pox.

☑ If you develop chicken pox at any time during pregnancy, discuss with your physician the possibility of using ultrasound to check for anatomical signs of congenital varicella syndrome.

☑ If you develop chicken pox within five days before delivery or two days after delivery, the Centers for Disease Control recommend giving your baby passive immunization with varicella-zoster immune globulin (VZIG). After two days, newborns and older infants who develop chicken pox should not have the immunization, as their risk of complications is no greater than is anyone else's.

CYTOMEGALOVIRUS (CMV)

Cytomegalovirus (CMV) is a member of the herpes family. It is very common in the general population. Around 80 percent of American adults have antibodies to CMV in their blood. This means most people have been previously infected by the disease and gotten over it, possibly without even realizing they were infected; it often has no symptoms and is only diagnosed by a blood test.

CMV is the most common cause of congenital viral infections in human babies. Most babies born with the infection express no signs of it at birth. When they do, these may include abnormalities of the blood, brain, and various organs. Some symptoms resolve themselves in time; others are serious or even life threatening. CMV causes about three thousand severely handicapped children in the United States each year. Once the disease is acquired, the baby usually continues to excrete the virus for months from its nose and throat and for years in its urine. Even babies without obvious illness at birth can, over time, develop complications, such as mental and neuromuscular defects and impaired vision and hearing.

• W H A T   T O   D O •

☑ Since most women have already developed antibodies to CMV, their unborn babies are not at serious risk from CMV infection, even if the mother comes down with the infection again. The greatest risk to the fetus occurs if a woman contracts CMV for the first time during pregnancy.

☑ If you need a blood transfusion during pregnancy or you or your newborn need one after delivery, the donated blood must be screened for CMV and be clear of the virus.

☑ One risky occupation for women attempting to become pregnant or already pregnant is providing day care. Being in intimate contact with large and changing groups of young children is a unique opportunity for exposure to a wide range of viruses, including CMV. Such providers and others exposed to groups of toddlers can have their blood checked for CMV antibodies. If they have antibodies, they do not have to worry about infecting their fetus. If they have never been infected, it is to their best interest to wash their hands frequently during the workday.

☑ Theoretically infants can become infected with CMV from breast milk, but experts say the health benefits of breast milk outweigh the possibility of the transmission of CMV infection to the infant.

FIFTH DISEASE

Fifth disease (erythema infectiosum) is one of the least-known infections of childhood. Its name is a carryover from a nineteenth-century method of categorizing diseases. The infectious agent is a virus, called parvovirus B19, which is a distant relative of the parvovirus found in dogs.

Fifth disease appears as a bright red rash on the child's cheeks (giving rise to its common name, "slapped cheek" disease) and a lacy rash across the body that can fade and reappear for weeks. Symptoms are so mild that no treatment is necessary, and the child may not appear ill until someone notices the rash. Since the virus is only contagious during the week before the rash appears, there is no reason to avoid contact with children who have the rash, for by this time they are no longer infectious.

The Centers for Disease Control in Atlanta have estimated that approximately half of all pregnant American women are already immune to fifth disease by the time they become pregnant, due to exposure during childhood. According to one study in the United Kingdom, few mothers who develop the disease pass it on to their fetus; when the fetus does contract it, there is no apparent risk of birth defects.

• W H A T   T O   D O •

☑ Nothing can be done. There is no commercially available blood test to find out whether or not you are immune. If you are pregnant, do not know your immune status, and someone you contact comes down with the disease, the CDC estimates your risk of miscarriage at less than 2.5 percent.

GERMAN MEASLES (RUBELLA)

German measles (rubella) is a viral infection that most often strikes children of grammar-school age in the spring and is usually quite harmless and mild. There is a rash, beginning on the face and spreading to the rest of the body, a low fever, tiredness, and perhaps some enlarged lymph glands. Adults may have additional symptoms, such as headache, aching joints, and higher fever.

In 1941 Australian ophthalmologist Sir Norman McAlister Gregg was the first physician to report that women who contracted rubella during the early months of pregnancy frequently delivered babies with one or more of three serious birth defects: cataracts, deafness, and a heart defect called ductus arteriosus (in which a blood vessel connecting the main pulmonary artery and the aorta remains open instead of closing, as is normal, within hours after birth).

Prenatal-rubella infection can also affect other organs and systems of the eyes, brain, skin, and bones. Certain abnormalities are not apparent until a year or two after birth, such as delayed language development, hearing defects, learning disabilities, and delayed motor development. Some researchers suggest that Type I diabetes (insulin-dependent) may be a delayed result of uterine exposure to rubella. The earlier in the pregnancy that the fetus is infected, the more severe the results, with a greater number of organs and systems involved.

During a rubella epidemic in the 1960s, some twenty thousand American children were born with severe problems. Thanks to widespread vaccination of schoolchildren, only one case of congenital rubella syndrome was reported in 1988—though others almost certainly occurred.

· W H A T   T O   D O ·

☑ Ideally, you will have had a blood test before pregnancy to determine if you are already immune to rubella. (If you had rubella as a child, you are usually immune for life.) If you are not immune and have not yet become pregnant, get immunized. If you are already pregnant and find out you are not immune, take care to avoid exposure to anyone who has been exposed to or diagnosed with rubella until you are well into your second trimester.

☑ It is extremely important that pediatric nurses and other hospital personnel who are pregnant (and not known to be immune to rubella) take precautions since a young child who was infected while in the womb can continue to infect others through contact with his body secretions and excretions up to several years past birth.

☑ If you need to get immunized, note that a committee of the Institute of Medicine of the National Academy of Sciences has found that one potential side effect of the rubella vaccine used today (RA 27/3) is acute arthritis. As always, you will need to discuss your individual situation with your physician as you plan your personal rubella-prevention program.

HEPATITIS B

Hepatitis B is a generally uncommon yet serious viral infection that can lead to chronic liver disease, cirrhosis, liver cancer, and premature death. The disease is especially prevalent among Alaskan Natives, Pacific Islanders, and people who abuse intravenous drugs or have sexual relations with intravenous-drug abusers. The virus is usually transmitted by exposure to infected blood or body fluids through punctured or broken skin and mucous membranes and by unprotected sexual relations with an infected person. It is not transmitted by casual contact.

Although the majority of adults recover and have lifelong immunity, from 5 to 10 percent are chronically infected carriers of hepatitis B and may continue to infect others. An estimated 850,000 to one million Americans are carriers. From 35 to 40 percent of the infants of carrier mothers become infected either at the time of birth or during infancy. In fact, a significant proportion of all hepatitis B is transmitted from mother to infant. The virus is not transmitted through breast milk.

The most obvious sign of hepatitis B infection is jaundice (a yellowish hue to the skin and the whites of the eyes). Other symptoms, which may develop slowly, are loss of appetite, nausea, vomiting, abdominal pain, skin rashes, and joint pain. A simple blood test reveals when the patient is infected with the virus and has the potential for transmitting the infection. About one out of every four children infected with hepatitis B virus around the time of birth will die prematurely of chronic liver diseases, such as cirrhosis or cancer.

As of 1991 Hawaii, New York, and California require doctors to test pregnant women for hepatitis B infection and to report every positive test result to the health department. This makes it possible to track the women so that their newborn infants can be treated in time to prevent damage.

· W H A T   T O   D O ·

☑ Women who need to be most concerned about hepatitis B are those who intend to travel widely in the Pacific Islands, Alaska, or other parts of the world where hepatitis B is prevalent or those who have contact with people from these areas. If you think you may be exposed to hepatitis B and your state does not require a blood test during pregnancy, make sure you are tested so if you do have the disease your newborn can be given the necessary treatment in time. Liver damage, cancer, or death are almost entirely preventable if the proper injections begin on the infected baby's day of birth and continue at one month and six months of age. These injections prevent chronic infection. The vaccine is very safe; side effects are rarely more than some tenderness and slight swelling at the site of the injections.

☑ Prevention of hepatitis B is best accomplished by maintaining a strong immune system and reducing exposure to the blood and body fluids of infected individuals. This includes avoiding direct contact with infected persons and accidental punctures from contaminated medical instruments. If you are a health-care worker and are not yet pregnant, experts advise vaccination.

☑ Even with a history of hepatitis B infection, new mothers can safely breastfeed.

HERPES SIMPLEX

According to the Herpes Resource Center, as many as 50 million Americans have cold sores caused by herpes simplex virus type I (HSV-I); approximately 40 million Americans may have genital herpes, which is usually caused by herpes simplex virus type II (HSV-II). From 200,000 to 500,000 new cases of herpes in people of all ages appear each year, with 1 newborn infected per every 3500 live births.

A sexually active person most often develops herpes of the genitals by engaging in sex with a partner who has an active infection. Although herpes type I usually originates on the mouth, a person can develop a herpes type I infection in the genital area after oral sex with someone who has a cold sore.

Herpes can be acquired and shed without any symptoms for months or years. This is of special concern to obstetricians, who want to protect babies from contracting the disease during birth.

In 1991 a report in the *New England Journal of Medicine* revealed that a mother's first-time infection toward the end of pregnancy leads to a risk of newborn infection much higher than previously realized. Most transmission from mother to infant occurs during delivery, when the baby's skin comes in contact with the virus-infected surfaces of the birth canal. If the doctor knows that the mother is shedding the virus, cesarean section will help protect the baby from herpes. Unfortunately, about 5 percent of infants develop herpes infections before delivery, due to viruses moving into the placenta from the mother's genitals. This transmission may be facilitated if an undiagnosed woman with herpes type II is electronically monitored (the insertion of electrodes into the fetus's scalp provides a means of entry for infection). In rare cases, a baby may be infected after birth from a mother with an oral or skin infection, or even from another infected baby in the hospital nursery.

Prevention of herpes infection in the newborn is extremely important, since as many as 80 percent or more of untreated infected infants will die. Blindness or other eye defects and brain damage are other common outcomes of neonatal herpes infection.

A woman who contracts herpes for the first time during pregnancy tends to have a more severe outbreak, sheds viruses for a longer period of time (an average of twelve days), and has lesions on her cervix in almost every case. She also tends to be at greatest risk of passing on the virus during delivery. Cervical lesions are especially dangerous, since it is there that the baby's face presses against an active sore.

If the woman has been infected prior to pregnancy but never had a visible genital sore, she sheds the virus for an average of eight days; the cervix is infected about 40 percent of the time. If the pregnant woman has had visible genital herpes infections before pregnancy, she sheds the virus for only about three days during the length of the attack; the cervix is involved only about 15 percent of the time, and she is least likely to pass on her infection to her infant. In addition, since she has been building up antibodies to the disease during years of infection and is bestowing these on her unborn child, she has been improving the infant's resistance to the disease.

· W H A T   T O   D O ·

☑ A Papanicolaou (Pap) smear or viral culture will reveal if you have an active infection during your last trimester. This will help your care giver decide on the safest method of delivery. It is not necessary to perform a cesarean section on every woman who has had a genital herpes outbreak during pregnancy. If laboratory cultures are negative repeatedly during the weeks prior to delivery, vaginal birth is considered safe.

☑ An inactive infection tends to become active during pregnancy. If you have ever had genital herpes outbreaks in the past, you must be especially careful to prevent an outbreak at this time.

☑ Eating nutritious meals is an excellent defense against herpes outbreaks. San Francisco general practitioner Richard Kunin, M.D., author of *Mega-Nutrition for Women* (New American Library 1983) recommends diets rich in betacarotene (orange-colored foods), vitamin B-6 (whole grains), and the mineral zinc (seafood).

☑ Avoiding oral-genital sexual contact during the last month of pregnancy is a good idea if either of you has a history of oral herpes infection. If the man has a history of herpes and the woman does not, pleasuring each other without intercourse during the last trimester is probably the safest route to take.

☑ Inform your obstetrician of any known history of herpes for either you or your mate so that your physician can search carefully for signs of infection. You may be infected but exhibit no symptoms until pregnancy brings them out in some subtle way.

☑ After delivery, keep anyone with cold sores or herpes sores anywhere on their body away from your newborn.

☑ For information on any aspect of herpes, contact the Herpes Resource Center Hotline, 919-361-2120 (9 A.M. to 7 P.M.) EST or get a copy of *The Truth about Herpes,* by Stephen L. Sacks, founder and director of the Herpes Clinic at the University of British Columbia, in Vancouver, Canada. If it is not available in local bookstores, order it from the Herpes Hotline, a service of the American Social Health Association, P.O. Box 13827, Research Triangle Park, N.C. 27709.

SYPHILIS

Syphilis is caused by a spiral-shaped bacterium named *Treponema pallidum.* The disease is contracted through intimate body contact with an infected person, including kissing a person who has a syphilitic lesion on his mouth. A single contact with an infected person creates a risk of infection of about 30 percent.

Unlike most diseases, syphilis appears in different forms at different stages. It first appears as a painless hard, wet ulcer called a chancre, which disappears. Months or even years later, the disease may progress to destruction of the heart, brain, and nervous system.

Untreated syphilis in the mother results in congenital infection in 75 to 95 percent of cases. Syphilis contracted in utero is life-threatening. Signs of infection in babies include premature birth, small size, and enlarged liver and spleen. When congenital syphilis manifests itself in later years, the children may show no symptoms; only a blood test reveals their condition. These children may remain symptomless until the third stage of the disease manifests during early adolescence. Only in about one-third of the cases in children over age two will youngsters show clear signs of disease, such as eye defects, nerve deafness, teeth and facial abnormalities, and skin defects. Several hundred cases of congenital syphilis still appear in the United States each year.

· W H A T   T O   D O ·

☑ Most women who arrange for prenatal checkups will automatically be given the blood test that detects syphilis. If you suspect you were exposed to the disease, arrange for such a blood test as soon as possible. You and your fetus can be treated simultaneously with penicillin. If the disease is of less than one year's duration, one injection is usually enough for a cure. For disease of longer duration, a weekly dose for three weeks is used. In addition, after delivery you and your newborn's cerebrospinal fluid will be checked to see if the disease has progressed to the central nervous system.

When a pregnant woman is treated during the first twenty weeks of pregnancy, there is rarely damage to her unborn child. Treatment later during the pregnancy or at birth will cure the infant's disease but cannot undo damage already done.

TOXOPLASMOSIS

If you have a cat who spends time outdoors or if you eat very rare meat, you could contract an infection called toxoplasmosis—named after the tiny protozoan *Toxoplasma gondii* that is its cause. Maternal toxoplasmosis can cause severe deformities in the fetus, especially when contracted during the first or early-second trimester. Luckily, at these stages the risk of a fetus acquiring the disease is smaller than later during the pregnancy.

Some of the problems associated with prenatal toxoplasmosis are hydrocephalus (water on the brain), small brain, convulsions, enlarged spleen and liver, and abnormally low blood count. Eye damage may occur but not be apparent for several years.

Toxoplasmosis is diagnosed in around 20 cases per 10,000 live births in the United States. Healthy adults almost always return to health without treatment and may not even realize they are infected; treatment of the fetus or newborn, however, is difficult, because effects can be so severe and there is no easy, safe drug to use.

· W H A T   T O   D O ·

☑ Prevent toxoplasmosis when possible. If you are planning to get pregnant or already are, stop eating very rare meat, especially lamb and pork. Never eat steak tartar or raw meat, and avoid meat that has been thawed and refrozen. Raw seafood is not a source of toxoplasmosis but may harbor other infectious agents and is not recommended.

☑ If you want to acquire a kitten, consider waiting until after delivery, as kittenhood is the peak age for contagion. If you already have a kitten, keep it indoors while you are pregnant. Cats that never kill rodents or other wild creatures are not ordinarily a source of toxoplasmosis.

☑ Since the major route of infection from cat to human is through cat feces, pregnant women owning outdoor cats should have others clean the cat box; be sure to have it cleaned daily. Days-old cat feces are most likely to harbor *Toxoplasma gondii,* so beware of encountering cat feces during gardening. Wear gloves.

Labor and Delivery

B y the time you have gone through pregnancy and reached the stage of labor and delivery, it may seem that there is nothing further you can do to prevent birth defects. In terms of the physical structure of the infant, that may be true. Since I, however, include long-term mental and emotional repercussions in my definition of birth defects, I will discuss labor and delivery practices that can affect the long-term well-being of the newborn. The following is a description of some of the most important interventions in labor and delivery that have been discussed in the medical literature.

INCOMPATIBLE BLOOD TYPE

About one Caucasian in six has Rh negative blood, meaning they are missing a substance on the surface of their red blood cells called the Rh factor; the term comes from the rhesus monkeys in which this factor was first discovered. Rh negative blood is rare in nonwhites.

When the mother is Rh negative but her first baby inherits Rh positive blood from the father, there is a 10 percent chance that before or during birth some of the baby's blood will intermingle with the mother's. This will cause the mother's body to produce certain antibodies. Then during a second or subsequent pregnancy with an Rh positive baby, those antibodies can attack and destroy the blood of the fetus. The new baby can suffer a form of severe anemia that can kill it or cause brain damage soon after birth unless treated by transfusion.

This chain of events is uncommon today, thanks to the widespread use of a vaccine called Rho (D) immune globulin—a commonly used commercial form is RhoGAM®. If an injection of this blood product is given to pregnant women who are Rh negative during their seventh month of each pregnancy, or within seventy-two hours after a miscarriage, abortion, or amniocentesis, a healthy baby can be born even in cases of blood-type incompatibility.

· W H A T   T O   D O ·

☑ Find out if you are Rh negative and if so, be sure to tell your obstetrician about abortions, miscarriages, and prior childbirths you have had at any time in your life—no matter how long ago. This information is important in designing a treatment plan to keep you and your newborn safe and well.

FETAL MONITORING

Electronic monitoring of the fetal heart rate is widely used to regularly monitor the fetal heartbeat during labor to identify any possible complications as early as possible. There are two types of electronic monitoring. External monitoring involves placing two straps around the mother's abdomen, one to pick up the fetal heart rate and the other to measure the intensity of contractions. Internal monitoring is more rarely used and involves passing a hooked wire through the mother's vagina and cervix, piercing the amniotic sac, and attaching the wire into the fetus's scalp to more directly monitor heart rate.

Although electronic monitoring is almost ubiquitous in some medical institutions, during the past fifteen years at least nine studies have revealed the procedure is of no greater benefit, even in cases of prematurity, than nurses doing the monitoring through handheld equipment, such as a fetoscope (an obstetric stethoscope) and a Doppler device (which measures soundwaves bounced back to the instrument from the fetus's bloodstream).

There are several important benefits of electronic monitoring. Some institutions with a shortage of nurses can have one nurse responsible for several machines at the same time. Continuous monitoring avoids the possibility of a nurse or physician missing important information should the fetus, by coincidence, be in trouble between the times of auscultation (listening with handheld devices). Additionally, an electronic device avoids the subjective interpretation by the auscultating nurse and, provided the equipment is adequately serviced, gives reliably objective data that is easily shown to colleagues for fast second opinions.

There are also several important drawbacks. Some research has noted higher rates of cesarean section among electronically monitored births. In addition, internal monitoring allows direct access along the lead wire to the infant's brain—an opportunity for herpes virus that may be in the mother's genital tract to infect the fetus. The Centers for Disease Control has found evidence linking such monitoring to herpes-related neonatal brain disease and death.

Both internal and external fetal monitoring limit the laboring woman's ability to walk around and take positions that make labor more comfortable and quicker. Thus, it can also contribute to the increased use of medication to enhance contractions, the use of forceps, and other forms of medical intervention that follow a lengthy labor.

· W H A T   T O   D O ·

☑ Find out in advance your doctor's and your hospital's position on fetal monitoring. Electronic monitoring became so popular so fast that it is currently considered standard medical practice. Consequently, if you wish to avoid the use of the equipment during labor, it is important that you make sure your hospital has adequate staff to personally monitor you and that your relationship with your physician is built on understanding and trust. To build that trust, you and your mate must accept responsibility for creating the kind of birthing experience you want and making your desires known. Be sure you also understand your physician's reasons for desiring to electronically monitor you.

☑ If electronic monitoring early in labor places you in the low-risk category, your physician may allow you to walk around to speed labor before again attaching you to the electronic monitor. The American College of Obstetricians and Gynecologists (ACOG) recommends that even patients at high risk may have nurse monitoring every fifteen minutes during the first stage of labor and every five minutes during the second stage—instead of continuous electronic fetal monitoring. For low-risk patients, ACOG advises using auscultation instead of fetal monitoring every thirty minutes in the first stage of labor and every fifteen minutes in the second stage.

DRUGS DURING LABOR

Many women are eager to use pharmaceuticals to make labor as quick and painless as possible. Other women are given drugs when they undergo cesarean section. In both cases, there are ramifications of drugs that you may wish to consider when preparing yourself for the birth experience.

Several studies have shown a direct relationship between the use of pain-relieving drugs and prolonged labor, leading to additional drug therapy to stimulate uterine contractions, medical intervention to withdraw the infant, abnormal fetal heart rates, and less-than-ideal Apgar scores (which does not necessarily indicate a permanent problem).

These outcomes are, in part, related to the laboring woman's confinement to bed once she is put on medication. Lying down means she is working against the force of gravity instead of with it, which slows down labor, making intervention more likely. When flat on her back, the pregnant woman's abdomen can also press down on major blood vessels, lowering her blood pressure and possibly reducing oxygen to the fetus.

Additionally, there are three other categories of drugs that may directly affect newborns: barbiturates, tranquilizers, and anesthetics. Near to delivery, barbiturates used to induce sleep or to reduce anxiety and fear in the mother can cause withdrawal symptoms in the infant and so-called floppy-baby syndrome. This involves feeding difficulties, shortened attention span, liver abnormalities, and other undesirable reactions collectively termed neonatal depression. Tranquilizers used on the mother, such as the benzodiazepines Valium®, Librium®, and Dalmane®, can cause lethargy, poor feeding, and poor temperature control; these conditions are undesirable for the infant and interfere with mother-infant bonding. In addition, tranquilizers may cause serious cases of jaundice.

Anesthetics used for labor and delivery can affect the school performance of children years after delivery. In testimony before the Senate Subcommittee on Health, Yvonne Brackbill, M.D., of the University of Florida, reported research concluding that anesthetics during labor can cause a slowing in the infant's motor development during the first year of life and, in later years, affect the development of language and thinking. General anesthesia produces stronger effects than local anesthesia, and local drugs result in more effects than no anesthesia at all. Given a need for surgery, the safest choice is regional anesthesia, using the smallest amount necessary of whichever drug will be eliminated by the body the quickest.

· W H A T   T O   D O ·

☑ An unmedicated birth is best. If you can, avoid the use of drugs that affect your labor and delivery.

CESAREAN SECTION

The use of cesarean section has increased during the past twenty-five years so precipitously that cesarean section has become the most commonly performed operation in the United States. At some institutions, one in three births is by cesarean.

Cesarean section is a major surgical procedure for the mother and results in more complications and risks than does vaginal delivery. The mother's risks involve reactions to the anesthesia and the possibility of infection, hemorrhage, and fever.

Cesarean-section babies are beautiful. They have none of the skull sculpting of babies pressed through the pubic bones, but they also have greater risk of hyaline membrane disease and other respiratory problems due to immature lungs. There is also increased risk of complications due to an immature liver and nervous system and to exposure to anesthetic drugs. Thanks to skilled prenatal diagnostic techniques and excellent medical care during and after surgery, however, infants born by cesarean section may have no side effects from their surgical grand entrance into the world.

The National Institutes of Health have attributed the sharp rise of cesarean delivery in the United States to three major causes: previous cesarean section, breech presentation of the fetus, and dystocia (meaning a difficult labor, including the so-called failure to progress). A discussion of each of these indications follows.

Vaginal birth after cesarean (VBAC).   In the 1960s and 1970s, it became increasingly common to perform a cesarean if a woman had previously delivered that way. By the 1980s, 99 percent of women who had given birth by cesarean had subsequent deliveries by cesarean.

Doctors automatically performed the operation because they feared that active labor would tear the scar from the first operation. Studies of vaginal birth after cesarean (VBAC) have proven this fear unwarranted in most cases. In fact, the American College of Obstetrics and Gynecology (ACOG) recognizes two important benefits of vaginal birth after cesarean: elimination of operative and postoperative complications and shortened hospital stay. Women who have had more than one cesarean have no greater risk of problems than women with only one previous cesarean. ACOG suggests that hospitals encourage women to have a VBAC, if there are no outstanding reasons why they should not go through labor.

Breech position.   A baby's position is breech when she arrives feet first. Cesarean delivery of breech babies has risen from about 12 percent in 1970 to about 79 percent in 1985, although studies have demonstrated no increased risk of trauma, cerebral palsy, or developmental delay in breech babies born vaginally compared to breech babies born by cesarean section.

Failure to progress.   Another common reason for cesarean section is called failure to progress, which includes two different labor problems. One is fear of infection if labor does not commence shortly after the bag of waters breaks. In the second, the cervix does not open adequately, although labor may have been hard and long.

Anxiety about motherhood, changes in a marriage or career, the tense atmosphere of some birthing environments, an ineffective or absent birthing coach, or even fear of making too much noise or of releasing a bowel movement can all decrease natural oxytocin, the hormone that stimulates uterine contractions. The woman may be unconscious of her high level of anxiety, and the less conscious she is, the more harmful the effects of anxiety may be to her and the fetus.

Failure to progress is a disappointing situation and makes you vulnerable for a cascade of interventions, beginning with intravenous oxytocin—Pitocin®. Because this therapy is delivered by an intravenous drip, it hampers your ability to change position or to walk around (walking around shortens labor by about 2.5 hours). Contractions stimulated by intravenous oxytocin can piggyback on one another, making relaxation between them difficult. Continuous fetal monitoring in bed further limits your mobility. If contractions become too forceful, an epidural will be used to relieve the increased discomfort or a muscle relaxant given to reduce the contractions. It is not unusual for this cascade to end with an emergency cesarean. In fact, failure to progress is the cause of almost one-third of all cesarean sections.

Children whose delivery was induced with oxytocin are more likely to need a special care unit, to be delivered with forceps, and to have breathing and sucking problems than uninduced infants. According to the Collaborative Perinatal Project, children exposed to oxytocin at birth had lower fine motor scores at age four and lower reading, spelling, and verbal-analogies scores at age seven. Statistics, of course, look at large numbers of deliveries, and within every group of babies that underwent difficult deliveries there are nevertheless some who grew up to be fine scholars and athletes.

· W H A T   T O   D O ·

☑ When you interview potential obstetricians, ask for the cesarean rates in their practices—and that of the hospital they will want you to use. If you have had a cesarean previously, discuss your desire for a VBAC. Be sure your obstetrician's expectations match your own.

☑ Since relaxation is a major key to making it through labor unmedicated, figure out ahead of time what might help you to relax. Some women decide to pursue meditation, biofeedback, or self-hypnosis training. If you are approaching this birth with many fears and tensions, read the chapter "Prematurity, Low Birth Weight, and Stress."

☑ Childbirth may be the most dramatic, physically demanding experience of your life, but you are equipped for it. What is invaluable is having a calm coach who helps you relax and reminds you to believe in yourself.

☑ Plan ahead. Drs. Marshall Klaus and John Kennell, whose research popularized the concept of parent-infant bonding at birth, have more recently introduced to Americans a useful concept that is practiced in other cultures; it lowers cesarean rates, shortens labor, reduces complications and fetal distress, and improves postpartum bonding. Sounds wonderful? It is as simple as having one consistent female companion throughout labor—a woman who has gone through it herself and is not taken aback by a laboring woman's drastic shifts in mood, demands, and fears. In Latin America this assistant is called a doula.

☑ The long-range effects of anesthesia are not inevitable or universal. If a cesarean may be necessary, discuss with your physician and anesthesiologist the medications that might be used and ways to minimize any known side effects.

☑ There are a number of techniques available to encourage a breech baby to turn head downward. One technique that your physician or midwife may try during the thirty-third to fortieth week of pregnancy is called external version. This entails rotating the baby by manipulating from the outside, through pressure on the mother's abdomen. The procedure must be performed by an experienced professional.

Alternately, Gayle Peterson, Ph.D., in *Birthing Normally* (Shadow & Light 1984) describes how hypnosis and visualization, using audiotapes you create for yourself, can affect the lower uterine nerves, allowing them to relax and expand, providing enough room for the baby to turn.

Another technique regularly employed in hospitals in China and in acupuncture clinics in the United States to turn a breech baby is called moxibustion. It involves warming a place on the foot the Chinese call *zhiyin* with a commercially prepared, smoldering stick of the herb mugwort (Artemisia vulgaris). In Chinese studies, this noninvasive, painless technique has corrected breech position over 90 percent of the time. Be sure to receive moxibustion from a licensed acupuncturist in a well-ventilated room.

☑ If your labor is active but not progressing and you have already been walking around, try stimulating your nipples. The benefit of this technique was scientifically proven in 1987 by physicians who measured the intensity and frequency of contractions (using an intrauterine pressure catheter) while women with ruptured membranes and absent or infrequent contractions stimulated their breasts.

☑ For publications or a sympathetic ear to listen to your feelings and fears, contact International Cesarean Awareness Network, Esther Zorn, President, P.O. Box 152, Syracuse, N.Y. 13210, 315-424-1942.

☑ Read the following guidebooks:

Visualization for an Easier Childbirth, by Carl Jones, (Meadowbrook 1988).

An Easier Childbirth, by Gayle Peterson, Ph.D. (Tarcher 1991).

Artemis Speaks: VBAC Stories & Natural Childbirth Information, by Nan Koehler. Order from N. Koehler, 13140 Frati Lane, Sebastopol, Calif. 95472 ($15 postpaid).

Open Season: A Guide to Cesarean Prevention and Vaginal Birth after Cesarean for the 1990s, by Nancy Wainer Cohen (Greenwood Press 1991).

The Expectant Parent's Guide to Preventing a Cesarean Section, by Carl Jones (Bergin and Garvey 1991).

PART THREE

After Pregnancy

Infant Feeding

Your child has arrived and with a lusty voice demands your full attention. You look with wonder at this miracle in your arms, so vulnerable, so needy, and you feel a sense of awe mixed with gratitude. How will you ever learn everything you need to know? Well, you will. And the information will come from many different sources. In fact, as you will quickly discover, even strangers will offer advice. Before you become totally intimidated, remember that no matter what you choose to do, someone is going to tell you how to do it better.

One topic that everyone seems to have a strong opinion on is infant feeding. You must make choices, and each carries with it consequences. This chapter examines food choices for the newborn and how they may affect the baby's health.

THE BREAST-FED BABY

Nature intended breast-feeding to be the perfect source of nutrition for your newborn. It provides a perfectly clean, digestible combination of fat, carbohydrates, protein, minerals, and vitamins at the perfect temperature without cost and available upon demand. Plus, if you tuck your baby next to you in bed or in a bassinet next to your bed, you never have to rise for 3 A.M. feedings.

Breast-feeding has been called the most elemental form of parental care, yet only about half the mothers in the United States are breast-feeding their infants by the time they leave the hospital. (When the statistics are analyzed by considering the mother's level of education, the figure rises: Fully 70 percent of college-educated women choose to breast-feed.)

Breast milk is one of the only sources for infants of DHA (docosahexaenoic acid), an omega-3 fatty acid that is important for good eyesight and optimum brain development. Breast milk also contains infection-fighting substances to help protect the newborn against bacterial and yeast infections. It eliminates the risk of baby-bottle syndrome (malformed jaws and poor dental development caused by juice or milk bottles left in the baby's mouth while it sleeps). According to the National Institute of Child Health and Human Development, breast-feeding also lessens the risk of Sudden Infant Death Syndrome by preventing gastrointestinal and respiratory illnesses. Other benefits include greater absorption of iron, less susceptibility to developing asthma and allergies during childhood, plus lower cholesterol and less likelihood of atherosclerosis in adulthood. Recent research has added to the long list of breast-feeding's benefits several others that last into adulthood, including reduced risk of inflammatory bowel disease and improved ability of body cells to grow and function to their full potential.

Your child can grow happily and healthily consuming breast milk as his primary source of food for the first six months of life. This is the recommendation of the Institute of Medicine's Food and Nutrition Board in a special report on breast-feeding published in 1991. Earlier than six months, the infant's digestive system is not ready to digest solids. If forced to eat solids, a young infant frequently develops food sensitivities and gastrointestinal distress.

The mother, too, benefits from breast-feeding. First, this special relationship between mother and infant grants an unparalleled level of intimacy. Second, the so-called letdown of milk that results from breast-feeding not only speeds the return of the uterus to its prepregnancy tone and dimensions but also enhances the mother-child bond through the influence of the hormone prolactin. You will also use calcium more efficiently, strengthening your bone mass and reducing your risk of osteoporosis. Breast-feeding, moreover, seems to reduce your risk of breast cancer.

Drugs and Chemical Hazards

The breast can be considered a magnificent device for delivering a pure product to the user, but it has no filter to eliminate impurities that may be circulating in your bloodstream and contaminating your milk. As a nursing mother you must continue to monitor, just as during pregnancy, your exposure to drugs and chemicals.

Unfortunately, even physicians may find it difficult to know whether any particular drug is or is not safe for a nursing mother. Many drugs have no supporting data that proves they are safe for pregnant or nursing women; the drugs may often be presumed safe simply because no one has reported adverse effects.

Drugs do enter breast milk. More blood flows into the breasts during lactation (milk production) than before pregnancy, and most drugs that are highly concentrated in the mother's blood diffuse into her milk. Drugs differ in the way they pass into breast milk, depending largely on the method of drug use (intravenous drugs concentrate in the milk the most quickly and in the highest levels) and the biochemical properties of the drug.

For example, one very important variable is a drug's solubility. Some drugs are soluble in the fat portion of the milk and some in the water portion. The milk an infant receives at the beginning of a feeding has less fat in it than the milk received at the end of a feeding. And the infant's first morning feeding has less fat in it than at midmorning, which is when fat is at its highest concentration. Thus, the amount of fat-soluble drugs that pass into the milk will vary depending on when the drug was taken, the dose, and whether it was instantly metabolized or gradually absorbed from a time-release capsule.

Once the drug or chemical is inside the infant, its effect depends on the ability of that unique individual to absorb it, metabolize it, and eliminate it. A baby's liver, kidneys, and other organs are constantly maturing, so she may be safe at two months from a drug that caused a side effect at one month.

Another issue related to the safety of breast milk is the mother's previous exposure to chemicals. Many dangerous substances are kept out of the bloodstream only because they are stored in fat cells. These substances include chlorinated and brominated pesticides, industrial chemicals, and dioxins. Women who have built up significant quantities in the fat in their breasts may release toxins into their milk during breast-feeding, as the fat is used up in the manufacture of milk.

In one widely publicized case, a six-week-old infant in Halifax, Canada, was poisoned by breast milk contaminated by the cleaning solvent perchloroethylene (PCE), which was inhaled by the mother when visiting her husband during lunch hours at his dry-cleaning job. The baby's liver disease improved after exposure to the solvent stopped. This is a poignant example of how breast milk can be a vehicle for hazardous substances.

Mercury and lead are two other environmental toxins that a nursing mother must diligently avoid. Unless your exposure to pollutants has been unusually severe, however, breast-feeding is still your best choice, since the ingredients of breast milk that improve the function of the infant's immune system are not available in any formula on the market today.

The following list includes the category, generic name, and one representative brand name of a few drugs that should not be used during breast-feeding. Be sure to check with your physician and pharmacist to learn of possible substitutes that might be less harmful than these drugs.

- Anticonvulsant: primidone, Mysoline®; phenobarbital, Bellergal-S®
- Antihistamine: clemastine, Tavist®
- Cancer remedies: cyclophosphamide, Cytoxan®, doxorubicin, Adriamycin®; methotrexate
- Diuretic: bendroflumethiazide, Naturtin®
- Immune suppressive agent: cyclosporine, Sandimmune®
- Migraine remedy: Ergotamine, Cafergot®
- Parkinson's disease therapy: levodopa, Larodopa®
- Prolactin suppressant: bromocriptine, Parlodel®
- Psoriasis remedy: Etretinate, Tegison®
- Stimulant: amphetamine, Dexedrine®
- Tranquilizer: lithium, Eskalith®

Several other commonly used drugs affect the nursing infant, for example:

Alcohol.   Mild use (one drink once in a while) by the mother may be harmless, but heavy use can lead to drowsiness, sweating, deep sleep, weakness, slowed growth, and abnormal weight gain in the baby—and decreased milk supply in the mother.

Antibiotics.   Most antibiotics are safe for the nursing mother and baby. Cyclosporine, however, should be avoided. The antibiotics erythromycin®; isoniazid, INH®, metronidazole, Flagyl®, tinidazole; and trimethoprim, Proloprim® might accumulate in breast milk if the mother is taking unusually high doses; the infant must be carefully monitored for signs of toxicity. With single-dose metronidazole therapy, discontinue breast-feeding for twelve to twenty-four hours. Sulfonamides (sulfa drugs) given to the infant during the first month of life can cause jaundice and may cause hemolytic anemia when given to the few children who have G6PD deficiency (a genetic enzyme-deficiency disease).

Caffeine.   An infant receives from your breast milk about 1 percent of your intake of caffeine, which might seem small. Some mothers, however, consume caffeine-containing beverages (coffee, tea, colas, hot chocolate) all day long, in addition to taking drugs that contain caffeine, such as Anacin®, Dristan®, and Midol®. Their infants can become hyperactive and wakeful—as would any adult stimulated by this drug.

Nicotine.   Smoking can reduce your milk supply. Exposing your infant to cigarette smoke increases the likelihood of allergies, hospital visits for childhood asthma and respiratory infections, Sudden Infant Death Syndrome, and lung cancer in later life. The baby's inhalation of second-hand smoke and consumption of nicotine from breast milk can cause shock, vomiting, diarrhea, rapid heart rate, and restlessness in the nursling. In addition, every cigarette she smokes reduces the mother's level of vitamin C and contaminates her and the baby with over 4000 different chemicals—many of which are carcinogenic.

Oral contraceptives.   Breast-feeding tends to suppress ovulation and helps to avoid a new pregnancy, but it is not reliable as birth control. Eventually, you will ovulate, and since that first period follows ovulation, you will not know when you are fertile. Since you can become pregnant while breast-feeding, regular use of reliable contraception is a good idea.

The American Academy of Pediatrics lists birth control pills as safe to take during breast-feeding, particularly the current low-dose formulations (using 30 mcg of estrogen in combination with progestin, or progestin alone). Since taking estrogens shortly after delivery can diminish milk supply, wait at least four weeks to begin using them. After that, the drugs will not change the quantity of your milk. They may, however, alter the composition of minerals, protein, and fat in it. Read the information found in the oral contraceptive package for a clear description of all the drug's ramifications. If you decide not to alter your natural hormone rhythms with the Pill, good alternatives are available. Call Planned Parenthood for details.

Painkillers.   Taking an aspirin (salicylates) or aspirin-containing pain reliever once in a while does not harm your breast-fed baby. If you are treating yourself for arthritis with more than 3 grams of aspirin per day, however, you may be altering your infant's platelets and, therefore, his body's capacity to form blood clots. The American Academy of Pediatrics lists aspirin among the drugs that have caused significant effects on some nursing infants and should be given to nursing mothers with caution. The AAP recommends measuring blood concentrations of aspirin in the infant when possible.

Radiology drugs.   The length of time that radioactive drugs remain in milk varies according to many factors, including dosage. It is important that you check with a medical specialist and even have your breast milk analyzed by a laboratory to make sure that the drug is gone before you resume nursing. Make sure that the nuclear-medicine specialist responsible for the test knows you are nursing, so you can be given a radionuclide that will disappear quickly from your milk.

Find out how long you will have to avoid nursing so that you can pump and freeze enough bottles of milk to feed the baby until you resume breast-feeding. Be sure to keep pumping and discarding milk during this time so that you maintain your milk supply.

It sometimes takes a few weeks for mother and baby to fall into an easy routine and rhythm. Nursing, at its best, is a relaxing, emotionally satisfying, and even sensual experience enjoyed equally by mother and baby.

THE FORMULA-FED BABY

By age two months, the majority of American babies are drinking formula. Some mothers, for a variety of physiological reasons (such as hormonal insufficiency, abnormal breast development, or previous breast-reduction surgery that included removal and replacement of the nipple) may not be able to breast-feed, no matter how motivated they are. Sometimes the infant, himself, has difficulty accomplishing proper nursing technique. Some women are in work situations that make continued regular breast-feeding impossible or choose to bottle-feed for other personal reasons. In such cases, a mother has a different set of choices: which formula to feed the baby.

Manufacturers of baby formulas usually include in their products everything they can that they know is essential for infant health; nonetheless, formula is not an exact replication of human milk. For example, there are no infection-fighting antibodies in formula. Also missing is the fatty acid DHA, the omega-3 fatty acid involved in development of the brain and the retina of the eye. To compensate for this lack, most liquid formulas contain soybean oil, a source of linolenic acid, which is an omega-3 fatty acid that the baby's body may be able to convert to DHA. (Note, however, that powdered formulas are often made with corn oil, which contains linoleic—not linolenic—acid. Linoleic acid interferes with the baby's ability to convert linolenic acid to DHA.) Formulas that are made with coconut oil (which is highly saturated and associated with cardiovascular disease) should be avoided.

In general, you can feel confident using a formula recommended by your doctor. During the late 1970s, however, one manufacturer of infant formula accidentally left out the element chloride from its two formulas, leading to significant developmental abnormalities and learning disabilities in the babies who were fed these products. To prevent this tragedy from recurring, Congress passed the Infant Formula Act, which gives the Food and Drug Administration the authority and the responsibility to make sure infant formula has within it everything a baby needs.

I am not a fan of formula, but I have to admit that my brother and sisters are all healthy, happy, and intelligent people—even though they were formula-fed. Breast milk may be best, but if your particular situation does not allow you to breast-feed, rest assured that loving nurturance can make up for what is missing in the bottle.

· W H A T   T O   D O ·

For mothers who choose to breast-feed their babies:

☑ The only medical reasons not to breast-feed are:

- acute (contagious) tuberculosis or acute cytomegalovirus (CMV)

- active hepatitis B

- human immunodeficiency virus (HIV)

- herpes simplex virus on the areola or nipple (a mother with herpes on the genitals or her mouth can still breast-feed)

- need for one of a very few medications that will harm the infant

- an addiction to cocaine, heroin, or other hard drugs (except methadone)

- galactosemia, a very rare genetic inability to digest milk
    Even mothers with a nonacute CMV infection and many with a history of breast cancer can safely breast-feed.

☑ The following organizations will answer questions about breast-feeding:
La Leche League, International
9616 Minneapolis Avenue
Franklin Park, Ill. 60131-7730
800-LALECHE or 708-455-7730 (Between 3 P.M. and 8 A.M. call 708-455-7730 for a volunteer mother who is on duty for nighttime emergencies.)

    Volunteers at LaLeche offer phone advice and organize meetings of breast-feeding mothers for free ongoing support and encouragement. Look in your local phone book under La Leche League for leaders near you.

International Lactation Consultants Association (ILCA)
201 Brown Avenue
Evanston, Ill. 60202
708-260-8874

    Lactation consultants are professional breast-feeding experts who help you overcome problems and recognize medical conditions that need attention. Obtain referrals to lactation consultants from ILCA, pediatricians, or childbirth preparation class instructors.

☑ Pay attention to your diet. A breast-feeding woman can become deficient in calcium, magnesium, zinc, folic acid, and vitamin B-6. While breast-feeding you need to consume 500 calories more than the amount needed to maintain your normal body weight and to drink plenty of water throughout the day.

☑ Consider alternatives to pharmaceuticals. Breast-feeding is so beneficial to the health of the infant that it is best for you and your physician to consider carefully whether prescribed drugs are absolutely essential and, if so, which will be least likely to affect your nursling. For example, before taking psychiatric medications for a severe case of postpartum depression ("the baby blues"), check to see if you have borderline deficiencies of B vitamins and minerals—such as calcium and zinc—that could be influencing your mental health.

☑ For more detailed information about the effects of medication on breast-fed babies, consult *Chemical Agents and Breast Milk*, edited by Judith Lauwers and Candace Woessner

(Avery Publishing Group 1990). Comprehensive lists of medications and other chemicals and their effect on the nursing infant are available from La Leche League International or from Breastfeeding Support Consultants, 164 Schoolhouse Road, Pottstown, Pa. 19464, 215-326-9343.

☑ When you take a drug the effect of which on the infant is unknown, be sure to ask your physician and pharmacist how you can calculte exactly when the drug will reach its greatest concentration and effectiveness in your body; then, alter your nursing schedule to reduce your baby's exposure to the drug. Generally, the best time to breast-feed is just before taking your medication, since it takes some time for drugs to move through the digestive tract and into the bloodstream. Also ask your physician and pharmacist about any signs of drug transfer to the infant. Babies can become ill from causes other than your medication.

☑ Prevent environmental pollution of your breast milk. If you work in an office or laboratory with volatile chemicals, search for ways to limit your exposure, such as moving your workstation or removing unnecessary sources of vapors. If you treat your home for insect infestation, hire an exterminator who uses a less toxic method than such chlorinated pesticides as chlordane, aldrin, or dieldrin.

Limit your consumption of food dyes, preservatives, and other sources of chemicals. Weigh your diet more heavily toward fresh or organically grown vegetables and grains. Reduce meat and dairy products, which concentrate environmental toxins. For adequate calcium, emphasize dark green leafy vegetables—such as broccoli, kale, and mustard greens—canned fish with edible bones, dried peas, beans, and citrus fruits.

☑ If you have reason to suspect you have been exposed to unusually high doses of drugs or toxic chemicals, you may want to have your milk analyzed. Ask your doctor to refer you to a test center and ask for an explanation of the results.

☑ Read *Total Nutrition for Breast-Feeding Mothers,* by Betty Kamen, Ph.D., and Si Kamen (Little, Brown 1986). You can order it from International Childbirth Education Association, P.O. Box 20048, Minneapolis, Minn. 55420,

800-624-4934. This book is an excellent reference guide, revealing not only the reality (compared to expectations) of the breast-feeding experience but also how to prevent contaminating your milk supply and how to solve common problems that mothers of newborns face.

For mothers who feed their babies formula:

☑ Your best choices are liquid formulas made with soybean oil, powdered formula to which linolenic acid has been added (Enfamil, Pro-Sobee, and Gerber's, for example), or powdered formulas that do not use corn oil and contain enough linolenic (S.M.A. and Nursoy).

Sudden Infant Death Syndrome

Sudden Infant Death Syndrome (SIDS) is the leading cause of death of infants from one month to one year of age. SIDS happens to about one out of every five hundred infants, most frequently between the first and fourth months and between midnight and 6 A.M. The tragedy is compounded because the death is not only sudden but is also unexplained—even after an autopsy, an examination of the site where the death occurred, and a review of the infant's medical history.

Although medical researchers still cannot name its cause, the following facts about SIDS are known:

- The risk of SIDS peaks at ten weeks and tapers off. It is very rare for a baby to die of SIDS before three weeks or after eight months of age.

- The rate of SIDS has not changed during the past forty years.

- The risk for SIDS is greater for males than females and for Afro-American and Hispanic infants than white infants.

- The incidence of SIDS drops in all populations as families improve their socioeconomic status.

- The risk for SIDS is higher among smokers and heroin and methadone users, and among premature babies and babies of low birth weight.

- The risk for SIDS is least in summer and greatest during winter but is similar in northern Canada and Southern California. It does not, therefore, seem to be affected by climate.

- There is no increased risk for a family that has already lost one child to SIDS.

- SIDS babies have more trouble than do other babies in clearing their lungs of foreign particles and have more inflammation of the respiratory tract. It has been suggested that indoor pollution affects the respiratory tract of SIDS babies more acutely than it affects that of other babies.

- A study conducted by the National Institute of Child Health and Human Development found that diarrhea and/or vomiting often occurred during the two weeks preceding SIDS. It is also common for SIDS babies to seem to be improving from what appeared to be little more than a common cold at the time of their death. The same study found that breast-feeding protected infants against SIDS and hypothesized that this protection may result from breast milk's ability to prevent gastrointestinal and respiratory illnesses.
- A number of epidemiological studies show a causal relationship between the pertussis vaccine and SIDS. Other studies show *no* causal relationship. Because immunizations of every kind are strongly encouraged by medical authorities, this relationship is highly controversial. Interested parents can contact the National Vaccine Information Center in Vienna, Virginia (703-938-DPT3), for more on the issue.
- Some SIDS babies seem to suffer abnormal heartbeat patterns.
- Infants dying of SIDS may have lower oxygen levels than normal infants or a lowered response to oxygen deficiency. A normal infant will wake up and cry when oxygen levels in the room drop. In one study, when oxygen levels were lowered, infants known to be at high risk of SIDS awakened later than low-risk infants.

Research indicates that early intervention may help prevent SIDS. In a British study, one group of mothers of high-risk infants were visited by a public-health nurse, who taught parenting skills, nutrition, and hygiene; she also showed the mothers how to recognize illness in their infants. A matched group received no postnatal visits. The group without postnatal education in parenting and nutrition had over three times the number of SIDS cases compared to the group visited by the nurses.

William Sears, M.D., is a pediatrician and author living in Southern California; he believes that if new mothers would breast-feed whenever their babies demand it and take their babies to bed with them, they could lower the risk of SIDS in their families. He encourages mothers to keep their babies close to their bodies as often as possible day and night.

In *Nighttime Parenting* (Penguin 1985), Sears explains that mothers and infants who sleep together begin to share REM sleep patterns. REM stands for Rapid Eye Movement and refers to eye motion that occurs during a period of deep sleep; it is considered the primary time during which dreaming takes place. Apparently, mothers and babies who sleep together actually dream simultaneously. Babies who are not suckled and kept next to the mother during the night do not show this coordinated dream pattern. Sears suggests that if, as some researchers suggest, babies dying of SIDS have more difficulty than normal in arousing themselves or have a deficiency of REM sleep, the stimulus of locking into the mother's REM pattern may help prevent SIDS.

Sears backs his enthusiasm for having the mother and infant share a bed with anthropological data showing the rate of SIDS approximately three to four times higher in cultures where babies are separated from their mothers during the night. Sears concludes his chapter on SIDS with this provocative question: "If there were fewer cribs, would there be fewer crib deaths?"

Position during sleep also seems important. Observant researchers noticed that Japanese mothers put their babies down on their backs at night, and Japan has one of the lowest incidences of SIDS in the world. In the Netherlands, Great Britain, and New Zealand, campaigns to convince mothers to lie babies on their backs have produced encouraging results. The Netherlands campaign began in 1987, and by 1988 crib deaths had dropped by 40 percent. The county of Avon, in England, found its incidence of crib death dropping by an astounding 51 percent the year and a half following a change in advice on infants' best sleeping position. Although it has not yet been proven that sleeping on the stomach is a *cause* of SIDS, it seems to be at the very least a contributing factor.

W H A T   T O   D O ·

☑ Handle the most obvious risk factors first, as follows:

- Get help to stop smoking or to kick a drug habit.
- Get in the habit of placing your baby on her back at night.
- If you can keep your infant out of childcare groups for her first six months, do so, suggests Bruce Beckwith, M.D., who has extensively researched SIDS. This avoids increasing the baby's chance of respiratory illness.

☑ Consider putting off immunizations until your infant passes the critical months for SIDS. Read *The Immunization Decision,* by Randall Neustaedter (North Atlantic Books 1991).

☑ For more information on the subject of SIDS, call or write to SIDS Alliance, 10500 Little Patuxent Parkway, Suite 420, Columbia, Md. 21044, 800-221-SIDS.

Your Child's Environment

W e parents have always had to protect our infants from environmental hazards. Centuries ago the dangers included burns from the cooking fire or poisoning from spoiled food, toxic plants, or contaminated water. Today there are new dangers (the water from our taps may contain chemicals instead of parasites), but it takes the same habit of alertness to keep our children safe as long as they are under our care.

In addition to alertness, we need knowledge, including what dangers exist and what to do about them. In this chapter, you will learn how to prevent organ dysfunction, immune system breakdown, frequent infections, allergic symptoms, and even cancer by making sure your child is not chronically exposed to hazardous substances during the first years of his life.

LEAD AND OTHER HEAVY METALS

Lead poisoning in children has been common since the 1920s. One of the most significant sources has always been lead paint. Today, it is estimated that 2 million children live in homes that harbor lead paint, where paint chips on the floor and in window wells are a continuous source of potential poisoning for crawling infants and toddlers. Lead particles from automobile exhaust or smelters may also accumulate in soil outside the home; it not only contaminates children playing outdoors but is also tracked into the house on everyone's shoes—thus contaminating infants and toddlers playing on rugs and floors indoors.

When researchers compared school performance and lead measurements in children's hair, a shocking picture emerged. The gifted children had the least lead; the normal, a quarter more lead; the low achievers, a quarter more than normal; and the very low achievers, ten times more lead in their hair than the gifted children.

Other toxic metals can affect learning ability. Researcher Dr. Charles Moon and associates studied children in the state of Wyoming and found extremely low levels of arsenic, mercury, cadmium, and aluminum linked to significantly poorer performance on academic tests compared to non-contaminated children.

· W H A T   T O   D O ·

☑ Take off your shoes when you enter the house. John R. Roberts, an engineer in Seattle, Washington, who has investigated lead abatement for the EPA, found that levels of lead in homes where inhabitants remove their shoes at the door are a fraction of that found in homes where people keep their shoes on. If shoe removal is not a practical option at your house, Roberts suggests you have everyone wipe the soles of their shoes twice on a thick industrial-quality mat at the door.

☑ Purchase lead-testing swabs from LeadCheck, P.O. Box 1210, Framingham, Mass. 01701 (800-262-LEAD) to test toys, floors, painted surfaces, ceramic glazes, food cans, and plumbing solder. Order their test for lead in water to test drinking fountains at your children's school. Some water fountains use lead-lined storage tanks.

☑ Test the soil outside your home for heavy metals. A soil test kit is available from Soil Testing Lab, West Experiment Station, University of Massachusetts, Amherst, Mass. 01003 ($7). If your soil is contaminated with lead, you may want to replace thick carpeting with small, easily cleaned rugs on wooden floors.

☑ Never sand or scrape off lead paint by yourself. Use an experienced contractor, relocate during home renovation, and do not return until postabatement testing proves the home is safe. One study found lead-dust levels up to six times greater and levels of lead in children's blood higher after abatement than before.

☑ What you can do is to wash home surfaces carefully, using trisodium phosphate (TSP, a detergent found in most markets and hardware stores). Learn the safest techniques for cleaning up lead by obtaining the fact sheet *Reducing Exposure to Lead in Older Homes*, by John Roberts. Send $1 to the Washington Toxics Coalition, 4516 University Way NE, Seattle, Wash. 98105, 206-632-1545.

RADIATION

Ionizing Radiation

American experts generally link radon only to lung cancer. In 1990, however, Denis Henshaw and colleagues at the University of Bristol looked at data from twelve nations and found that childhood cancers of the brain, spine, bone, and skin (melanoma) were also linked to radon exposure.

Nonionizing Radiation

Dr. Nancy Wertheimer, of the University of Colorado Medical Center, published a pioneering study in 1979 on the effect on children of living in homes near overhead high-current power-transmission lines. Wertheimer found twice the rate of leukemia, lymph node cancer, and nervous-system tumors in the homes near high-current lines as in nearby homes near low-current lines. These study results were redone on a larger scale by Dr. David Savitz in 1988; he also found that exposure to electric-power distribution lines was associated with higher rates of childhood cancer.

· W H A T   T O   D O ·

☑ Read "Environmental Toxins" for specific suggestions on testing your home for radon and on reducing exposure to nonionizing radiation.

CIGARETTES

Nicotine is one of the major drugs to which infants and young children are exposed. Switching to a low-tar brand may increase the risk to your baby, since second-hand smoke from low-tar varieties contains up to 30 percent more cancer-causing substances than do the high-tar brands. Children of smokers suffer brain cancer 50 percent more often than do children of nonsmokers. They also suffer other forms of cancer in greater numbers.

Infants of smokers are at greater risk than infants of nonsmokers of dying from Sudden Infant Death Syndrome. Young children in the home of smokers are at higher risk of developing inner-ear infections, bronchitis, and pneumonia—especially if both parents smoke. The greater the number of cigarettes smoked in the house, the greater the number of respiratory infections in the infants living there. Children of smokers are often shorter than children of nonsmokers, and they are poorer readers.

· W H A T   T O   D O ·

☑ Quit smoking. Read "Recreational Drugs" for specific suggestions to help you and your mate quit. At the least, do not smoke in your house or car.

CHEMICALS AND PESTICIDES

Household chemicals, such as drain and oven cleaners, and pesticides are acutely toxic; they can damage an infant or small child after only one exposure. Other household chemicals cause chronic toxicity, leading to a breakdown of the child's immune system, chronic infections, autoimmune diseases, allergies, or cancer.

Infants are particularly vulnerable to chemical contamination, yet we may unwittingly prepare a special room for them loaded with chemical-soaked fabrics and furniture that continuously release poisons into the room. For example, formaldehyde frequently outgasses from particleboard, plywood, carpeting, draperies, and permanent-press linens, causing respiratory symptoms, skin disorders, and possibly, over years of exposure, even cancer. Other chemicals reach the infant from aerosols, air fresheners, carpet backing, dry-cleaned clothes, and cleaning products.

The agricultural use of pesticides is increasingly suspected of causing long-term health problems. Studies done in Finland found cancer more frequently in children whose mothers lived on a farm or whose fathers worked in agriculture, gardening, or forestry—all professions where pesticide exposure was probable. Additionally, neurotoxins in pesticides influence how the brain functions. According to the Congressional Office of Technology Assessment, "research demonstrates that pesticide poisoning can lead to poor performance on tests involving intellectual functioning, academic skills, abstraction, flexibility of thought, and motor skills; memory disturbances and inability to focus attention; deficits in intelligence, reaction time, and manual dexterity; and reduced perceptual speed. Increased anxiety and emotional problems have also been reported." The National Academy of Sciences suggests that 12 percent of the children under age eighteen in the United States have mental disorders; it claims that toxic exposures before and after birth contribute to the creation of these problems.

Pesticides are especially dangerous because they are not usually tested for their effect on young children. According to Anne Witt Garland, in *For Our KIDS Sake* (Sierra Club Books 1989), "if all of today's preschoolers were exposed at the maximum levels permitted by the EPA to just three fungicides—captan, folpet, and mancozeb—more than 20,000 children could eventually develop cancer during their lives as a result of that exposure during their preschool years alone."

· W H A T   T O   D O ·

☑ Read labels. This is the best way to learn which products have toxic ingredients. Does the label warn about using proper ventilation or eye protection? These are good clues it contains poisons that you want your newborn to avoid.

☑ Use nontoxic alternatives instead of chemical-laden products. For example, use pine or other solid-wood furniture, not particleboard; open windows instead of using air fresheners; and use baking soda, borax, salt, white vinegar, and lemon juice for household cleansers. Since bleach fumes mix with the moist air in laundry rooms and form hydrochloric acid (which irritates the respiratory tract), keep your infant or toddler in another room if you insist on using bleach.

☑ Call the Chemical Manufacturer's Association (800-CMA-8200) for information about the chemicals found in specific consumer products. Since formaldehyde outgassing lessens with the age of the product, used plywood or pressboard furniture is safer than new products. You can also stop outgassing by sealing products with a water-based or polyurethane sealant.

☑ Use multiple layers of clothing and a warm head covering on your infant instead of placing an unvented gas or kerosene space heater near the crib. This protects the baby from poisonous combustion gases, such as carbon monoxide, nitrogen oxide, and sulfur dioxide. Alternately, vent the heater to the outside or use an electric heater.

☑ To excellent sources of information on alternatives to pesticides are:

Bio-Integral Resource Center, P.O. Box 7414, Berkeley, Calif. 94707 (415-524-2567). It offers material on safe, natural pest management methods. Write for a free information packet.

Washington Toxics Coalition, 4516 University Way NE, Seattle, Wash. 98105 (206-632-1545). WTC offers excellent fact sheets on safer household and household-cleaning products, home and garden pest management, and lawn care. (Cost: $1 each or all fourteen for $8.)

☑ See more suggestions on preventing pesticide contamination in "Environmental Toxins."

☑ Two excellent books have recently been published to help parents identify dangerous chemicals in their home and create an oasis of safety for their family:

The Nontoxic Baby: Reducing Harmful Chemicals from Your Baby's Life, by Natural Choices (204 North El Camino Real, Apartment E214, Encinitas, Calif. 92924 ($9.95, plus $2 shipping). A group of parents created this spiral-bound handbook (literally, it fits in your hand) to give consumers the briefest outline of information on dangerous chemicals and how they may be affecting your baby in the bedroom, in babycare products, or in food or drink.

Poisoning Our Children: Surviving in a Toxic World, by Nancy Sokol Green (Noble 1991). Green shares her story of pesticide and formaldehyde poisoning in her own home, how she created a safe home for her family, and how others can discover and eliminate health hazards that endanger their young children.

Afterword

I t would have helped you if I had been able to create a rating that showed the approximate risk inherent in each hazard mentioned in this book. When I asked an environmental scientist who works for the EPA about doing so, he explained how very difficult that would be, given our present lack of knowledge about the reproductive effects of so many factors in our environment.

We must accept the fact that as we attempt to prevent birth defects at the dawn of the twenty-first century we are working with a great many unknowns. We are all pioneers in this effort—researchers, physicians, and parents-to-be alike. I hope that in reading this book and learning what might help create a successful pregnancy and healthy child, you have discovered that in spite of the scary prospect of leaping into the unknown, you do have control over a great many variables connected with birth defects. Much can be accomplished without enormous difficulty or expense; sometimes the simplest changes can be the most profound.

After a year and a half of research on this topic, I offer you my own Top Ten priority list for those changes, in the order of their importance:

1. Follow the preconception self-care program developed by Foresight (p. 2324).

2. If you have diabetes, get help maintaining control of your blood sugar before you become pregnant and during your pregnancy. Even if you don't have diabetes, obtain prenatal care.

3. Every day, before and during pregnancy, eat nutrition-rich foods, especially a wide variety of vegetables and whole grains such as 100 percent whole-wheat products and brown rice.

4. Take prenatal nutritional supplements before conception and continue them through pregnancy.

5. Stop drinking any alcoholic beverage before conception and continue to avoid all alcohol during pregnancy.

6. Under your doctor's supervision, stop all pharmaceuticals before conception and through the entire pregnancy and labor.

7. Stop smoking cigarettes before conception and do not allow anyone else to smoke in your presence during your pregnancy or in your home when your child is present.

8. Before, during, and after pregnancy, both parents avoid unshielded exposure to potentially hazardous substances like chemicals and ionizing radiation.

9. Before, during, and after pregnancy, get help releasing yourself from an addiction to mind-altering drugs.

10. Breastfeed your newborn for at least four months (which takes you over the painful phase and into sheer pleasure).

If you write to me, I can share in future editions of this book your personal story, and others will benefit from the efforts you have undertaken to prevent birth defects before, during, and after your own pregnancy. Thanks!

Carolyn Reuben
c/o Jeremy P. Tarcher, Inc.
5858 Wilshire Blvd., Suite 200
Los Angeles, Calif. 90036

The Most Common
Birth Defects

The following is an alphabetized list of some common or well-publicized structural birth defects, and the frequency of their occurrence in the general population.

Anencephaly—3 per 10,000 births

Anencephaly refers to the absence of the brain due to lack of development of the neural tube—the part of the embryo that becomes the brain and spinal cord. The condition may be discovered prenatally by maternal blood test, ultrasound, or amniocentesis. Much research suggests some neural tube defects might be caused by maternal deficiency of folic acid and other nutrients and prevented by preconception and prenatal vitamin supplementation.

Birthmarks—1 per 3 to 4 births

A birthmark is an area of discolored skin apparent at birth, such as moles or hemangiomas. Moles are abnormal deposits of dark pigment and may be removed by plastic surgery later in life.

Hemangiomas are abnormalities of blood vessels that cause strawberry marks (raised areas that usually fade by age seven) or port-wine stains (flat, large areas that can be removed by laser during childhood).

Cerebral palsy—2 to 6 per 1000 births

Cerebral palsy involves brain damage that more often affects the area of the brain controlling motion than the area used for thinking. Thus, muscles of one or more limbs and often other parts of the body are rigidly contracted (or, less commonly, flaccid or writhing), making smooth movements difficult or impossible. Depending on severity and which limbs are involved, the child may learn to walk. In some cases, the child is mentally retarded, but it is common for children with cerebral palsy to be very intelligent. The condition can include hearing loss, speech impediments, crossed eyes, and convulsions. Cerebral palsy is not hereditary and does not worsen over time. With skilled therapy, both movement and speech can improve. Many children with cerebral palsy grow up to lead independent lives.

Cleft lip—*1 per 1000 white births and 1 per 2500 Afro-American births*

Cleft lip involves incomplete closure of the upper lip on one or both sides, resulting in a vertical split that may extend to the nose. The condition was once called hare lip, but this term is no longer used because it is both inaccurate and insulting. Cleft lip is usually corrected by surgery in infancy and may or may not be associated with cleft palate. When the cleft is combined with a single upper tooth or the absence of the vertical groove between the lip and nose, it may indicate what is called a central midline defect, which is often associated with brain damage. Nutritional deficiencies and home pesticide use have both been implicated by various studies as possible causes of this problem. Since the lip is completely formed by the end of the fifth week after conception, any drug or environmental toxin the mother was exposed to after her fifth week cannot be a cause of this condition.

Cleft palate—*1 per 1500 births*

Cleft palate is the incomplete formation of the roof of the mouth. It may or may not be associated with cleft lip. It is usually surgically corrected at around one year of age; the child may still need further repair at a later date in addition to speech therapy. The palate is basically formed by the end of the seventh week following conception, so any drug or environmental toxin a mother was exposed to after her seventh week of pregnancy cannot be to blame for this condition.

Club foot—*1 per 1500 births*

In club foot, the foot or feet are abnormally twisted, usually with the heel inward and the foot downward and inward. If treated before age two, the child may walk normally. Treatment may involve manual manipulation, a plaster cast, splinting, taping, or surgery, depending on the severity and age of the child when treatment begins.

Congenitally dislocated hip—*1 to 2 per 1000 births*

Instead of sitting neatly in its socket in the pelvic girdle, the ball-shaped top of the thigh bone may be out of place in one or both hips. Dislocated hip occurs most frequently in girls and tends to run in families. It is often discovered at birth and is treated by a soft cloth sling for six to nine months. If treated early, the child will walk normally. If not, major hip surgery may be needed later in life.

Cystic fibrosis—*5 per 10,000 births*

Cystic fibrosis is a hereditary defect mainly affecting the lungs and intestines. The child's lungs produce a thick, sticky mucus that is not coughed up and leads to frequent bouts with pneumonia and other respiratory infections. The child's pancreas does not produce digestive enzymes, so nutrients are not absorbed from the intestines. Antibiotics fight the infections, and nutritional supplements and digestive enzymes help prevent malnourishment, allowing children to live into adulthood. Scientists have been able to identify the exact gene responsible for this condition, which means there may be significant therapeutic advances in the near future.

Digestive tract atresias
  Esophagus—1 per 32,000 births
  Intestines—1 to 4 per 20,000
    births
  Bile   *—1 per 8000 to 10,000*
    births

The term *atresia* means one or more segments of the digestive tract are missing, creating dead ends where a continuous opening should be. Common sites are the esophagus, bile ducts, small intestine, or anus. Intestinal atresia is diagnosed in the newborn by such symptoms as lack of bowel movements, an abdomen swollen with gas, and regular vomiting of green colored bile (a digestive juice produced by the liver). Any newborn vomiting green material must be brought immediately to the pediatrician for an examination, as an atresia diagnosed early enough can usually be corrected with surgery.

Down syndrome—*Incidence varies by mother's age. See table 7.*

Down syndrome is a genetic condition of mental retardation and characteristic facial and bodily features due to the presence of an extra chromosome number 21. Down syndrome is also called Trisomy 21, referring to the presence of a third (*tri*) chromosome. The condition is no longer called mongolism.

Down syndrome is usually caused by defective chromosome distribution during egg or sperm formation. This means the woman's egg was damaged while she, herself, was still an embryo, or, in about 20 percent of cases, the father has contributed a damaged sperm.

In about 4 percent of cases, Down syndrome results from one chromosome breaking and attaching to another chromosome within an egg or sperm or, also rarely, from faulty distribution of chromosomes in cells of the child itself while still an embryo. These vents may be caused by environmental factors, such as occupational exposure to microwaves, but such cases are not widely documented.

Down syndrome occurs in all socioeconomic groups. For an unknown reason, more males than females are born with this condition. Children of parents over age forty are at particular risk, but actually 80 percent of children with Down syndrome are born to women under age thirty-five, due to the greater number of women of this age group having children.

Retardation due to Down syndrome varies from very mild to severe. The children often have health problems, including heart and intestinal defects, greater susceptibility to ear infections (causing hearing and speech problems), respiratory conditions, leukemia, premature aging (after age thirty-five), and Alzheimer's-like symptoms of dementia. Life expectancy is around fifty-five years of age.

Table 7. Incidence of Down syndrome by age of mother

Incidence	Age of Mother
1 per 2000 births	20
1 per 1400 births	23
1 per 1000 births	29
1 per 800 births	31
1 per 600 births	33
1 per 400 births	35
1 per 300 births	36
1 per 200 births	38
1 per 110 births	40
1 per 30 births	45

Fragile X syndrome—.5 to 1 per 1000 births

Fragile X syndrome is an abnormality on one section of the X chromosome that is carried by mothers and inherited most often by their sons. About 80 percent of boys with fragile X syndrome are mentally retarded. Common physical features include long, narrow faces; prominent ears, forehead, and jaw; and enlarged testicles. Hand-slapping or hand-biting is also common.

Gastroschisis—8 per 100,000 births

Gastroschisis is an opening in the wall of the abdomen that allows abdominal organs, especially the intestines, to protrude out of the body. Prenatal testing often can identify this problem, which, in some cases, may be solved with relative ease by surgery soon after birth.

Heart defects—1 per 100 births

Many heart defects are minor and require no therapy, such as some heart murmurs (abnormal sounds). Even some holes spontaneously close, in time. Serious defects require surgical correction. The parent may first notice poor appetite and growth, little energy, breathlessness, and bluish coloration of nails, lips, and skin. In some cases, surgery is best done before the child is five; in others, before the child is ten. Names of some common heart defects, in which abnormal connections, holes, or narrowings occur in various parts of the heart, include tetralogy of Fallot, patent ductus arteriosus, transposition of the great vessels, and atrial or ventricular septal defect.

Hydrocephalus—1 per 2000 births

Hydrocephalus (water on the brain) involves excessive cerebrospinal fluid within the brain's hollow spaces, expanding the brain and often enlarging the head's circumference. It has various causes, including a maternal viral infection or fetal hemorrhage (which may itself be due to an impaired ability of blood to clot due to prematurity). If untreated, brain damage usually results. By placing a permanent shunt in the baby's brain, it is possible to drain off fluid into the lower body, allowing the head to return to average size and offering the child a good chance at normal development.

Hypospadias—3 per 1000 male births

Hypospadias is the existence of one or more openings on the underside of the male newborn's penis. It is often associated with other genital defects, such as undescended testicles or hooded foreskin. The condition is surgically corrected during the first two years of life and usually allows the boy to urinate normally and, as an adult, to enjoy normal sexual intercourse.

Lactose intolerance
97 per 100 Thai
87 per 100 Chinese
80 per 100 Native Americans
70 per 100 Afro-Americans
50 per 100 Hispanics
20 per 100 Caucasians

Around 70 percent of the world's adult population are deficient in an enzyme called lactase, which allows humans to digest lactose, the form of sugar in milk. The minority of people who have this enzyme are mostly descended from milk-drinking northern Europeans and nomadic herders in Africa and the Middle East. In contrast to most inherited birth defects, lactose intolerance is actually the original condition of humans, with the ability to digest milk into adulthood originating by genetic mutation. Symptoms of deficiency include diarrhea, vomiting, stomach cramps, gas, and eczema. Adequate calcium can be obtained by breastfeeding and then using calcium-rich vegetables, nuts, and seeds.

Muscular dystrophy—*1 per 3500 boys, most common form*

Muscular dystrophy involves slow, progressive degeneration of muscle fibers. More than forty forms exist. The most common and well-known form is called Duchenne muscular dystrophy. In about 95 percent of cases, boys inherit Duchenne's from their mothers, who are carriers. Occasionally, the disease occurs, instead, due to an unexplainable genetic mutation. Duchenne's is usually diagnosed around age five, but other forms may not manifest until the child is in his or her teens or early twenties. There is no known effective treatment, but new research is promising. Muscular dystrophy is detectable through prenatal testing. Siblings of any child with the condition can discover if they are carriers through a blood test (which is most reliable if taken before puberty).

Omphalocele—*2.4 per 10,000 births*

Omphalo- relates to the navel; *-cele* means herniated. With omphalocele, the intestine and sometimes other abdominal organs protrude through the navel covered only by a thin membrane. Prenatal testing can often diagnose this problem. It is not unusual for omphalocele to be associated with other birth defects, including chromosome abnormalities. If there is no other defect, the baby can be treated successfully by surgery.

Phenylketonuria—*1 per 16,000 births*

Phenylketonuria (PKU) is a rare inherited absence of the enzyme that converts the amino acid phenylalanine into another amino acid, tyrosine. It is extremely important for a woman with phenylketonuria to lower her phenylalanine levels before she becomes pregnant and if her child has the disorder to avoid feeding the child many phenylalanine-rich foods, such as milk or meat; otherwise, the amino acid will accumulate in the child's body and cause mental retardation. Ninety percent of PKU patients are blond and blue-eyed. PKU is diagnosed by a blood test. Associated conditions include seizures, so-called mousey body odor, and eczema.

Polydactyly—50 per 100,000 births

The term *polydactyly* means excessive fingers or toes. They may be fully formed, stuck together with other digits, or appear as ill-formed rudimentary stumps. The condition sometimes runs in families. Extra digits are usually removed surgically.

Pyloric stenosis—1.6 per 1000 births

With pyloric stenosis, the walls of the passageway from the stomach to the small intestine are thickened, and the opening is so severely narrowed that the baby's stomach must contract violently after every feeding to squeeze some food through. This backfires, as the force projects food up the esophagus and out the infant's mouth—sometimes several feet in the air. The baby (often a first-born male) is chronically hungry, anxious, and biochemically imbalanced. The problem is completely corrected by surgically opening the passageway. Nutritious feedings are important once food stays down.

Sickle-cell anemia—150 per 100,000 Afro-American babies

Sickle-cell anemia is an inherited blood disorder carried as a recessive gene by 1 in 12 Afro-American adults. Normally round, flexible red blood cells become stiff and sickle-shaped, reducing their mobility and hastening

their destruction. Most sufferers are Afro-American, but some are from Mediterranean, Middle Eastern, and southern Asian countries.

People who have inherited the gene from only one parent do not have the disease, but are carriers. Six or seven out of every 1000 Afro-American couples are both carriers; together they can pass the disease on to their children. Children with the condition are at risk of infections, bone pain, and damage to various internal organs. Painful blocked blood vessels or other serious symptoms (including heart attack, kidney failure, and stroke) may develop after an injury, under anesthesia, during infections, or during times of low oxygen, such as during airplane travel or even just at mountain altitudes. Also, all the usual symptoms of anemia will develop, such as weakness, tiredness, and heart palpitations. There is no known cure. Pregnant women and children with sickle-cell anemia are helped by blood transfusions and preventive antibiotics. Carrier status may be diagnosed by a blood test, and prenatal testing can determine whether a fetus has the disease.

Spina bifida—1 per 1000 births; 5 per 100 for women with 1 affected child

Spina bifida is categorized as a neural tube defect and involves incomplete closure of the spinal column around the spinal cord. Resulting disabilities vary widely from mild to severe loss of bladder, bowel, and lower-limb control to loss of life. A mother's use of drugs, such as valproic acid (used to control seizures) or retinoic acid (a derivative of vitamin A), have been implicated in some cases. Several studies show that the use of a vitamin supplement containing folic acid, among other nutrients, during the first six weeks of pregnancy, can reduce the risk of spina bifida by as much as 74 percent.

Tay-Sachs Disease—*1 per 3000 to 3500 pregnancies among Ashkenazic Jewish couples*

Tay-Sachs Disease is a deficiency of an enzyme called hexosaminidase A; it results in abnormal brain biochemistry, leading to blindness, dementia, paralysis, seizures, and deafness, with death occurring during the first few years of life. This disease strikes Jews of Ashkenazi (Eastern European) descent 100 times more often than people of other ethnic groups. In the past twenty years, the incidence among Jews has sharply declined to the point that barely ten cases appear in the United States per year, probably due to greater use of preconception and prenatal testing. A simple blood test reveals carrier status.

Thalassemia—*unknown rate of occurrence*

Beta thalassemia, according to the March of Dimes, is uncommon but not rare. As with sickle-cell anemia, thalassemia is due to an inherited abnormality of hemoglobin in the red blood cells, leading to weakness, tiredness, paleness, and breathlessness.

People who carry a defective gene inherited from only one parent have beta-thalassemia minor and suffer only minor symptoms. A pregnant woman who is a carrier, however, may develop temporary anemia as a result of biochemical changes during pregnancy.

If a child inherits a defective gene from both parents, the child develops beta-thalassemia major (formerly called Cooley's anemia) and needs repeated blood transfusions to stay alive. The transfusions cause an excess of iron, which necessitates chronic drug therapy to prevent liver or heart failure.

Resources

HOTLINES

The following hotlines offer information about genetics, drugs, chemicals, and other environmental agents that might damage a fetus or infant. In some cases you will be given the information you need immediately. In many others, you will have to wait for someone to find the answer to your question and call you back. Technically these are not hotlines but, rather, risklines. Most hotlines and risklines are run by universities or hospitals and serve only residents of their own state or region. If your state is not listed below, call the national hotline number or a local March of Dimes office for a referral.

NATIONAL

Environmental Safety Council of New York City runs this nonemergency service, which will refer you to a local environmental agency in your state that will be able to answer your questions.
800-2-TEST ME.

ARIZONA

Arizona Teratogen Information Program/Arizona Health Science Center, Tucson
800-362-0101, 602-626-6016

ARKANSAS

Arkansas Genetics Program—
Preconception Counseling
501-686-5994

Genetics Program Teratogen Screening/University of Arkansas for Medical Sciences (Little Rock)
501-686-5994 (for health-care professionals only)

CALIFORNIA

Teratogen Registry/University of California, San Diego
800-532-3749, 619-294-6084

COLORADO

Teratogen Information Program at
    Children's Hospital (Denver)
800-332-2082, 303-861-6395

CONNECTICUT

Pregnancy Exposure Information
    Service/University of Connecticut
    Health Center (Farmington)
800-325-5391, 203-679-1502

FLORIDA

Division of Genetics/University of
    Florida (Gainesville)
904-392-4104

Teratogen Information Service/
    Department of Pediatrics/
    University of Miami School of
    Medicine (Miami)
305-547-6464

Teratogen Information Service/
    Department of Pediatrics/
    University of South Florida
    (Tampa)
813-974-2262

ILLINOIS

Teratogen Information Service Office
    of Genetics/Illinois Masonic
    Medical Center (Chicago)
800-252-4847, 312-296-7095

IOWA

Department of Pediatrics, Medical
    Genetics/University of Iowa
    (Iowa City)
319-356-2674

MASSACHUSETTS

Pregnancy Environmental Hotline/
    National Birth Defects Center/
    Franciscan Children's Hospital
    (Boston)
800-322-5014, 617-787-4957

MISSOURI

Genetics Department, Department of
    OB-GYN/Washington University
    School of Medicine (St. Louis)
314-454-8172

MONTANA

Pregnancy Riskline/Utah State
    Department of Health (Salt
    Lake City)
800-521-2229 (Montana)

NEBRASKA

Teratogen Project/University of
    Nebraska Medical Center (Omaha)
402-559-5071

NEW JERSEY

Teratology Information Network/
    University of Medicine and
    Dentistry of New Jersey (Camden)
609-757-7869
    Residents of New Jersey interested
in printed material about occupa-
tionally related reproductive and other
health issues can contact The Resource
Center of the Environmental and Occupational Health Information Program, Division of Consumer Health
Education, Department of Environmental and Community Medicine,

UMDNJ-Robert Wood Johnson Medical School, Brookwood II, 45 Knightsbridge Rd., Piscataway, N.J. 08854.

NEW MEXICO

Department of Obstetrics and Gynecology/University of New Mexico (Albuquerque)
505-272-6391 (New Mexico residents)

NEW YORK

Western New York Teratogen Information Service/University of New York at Buffalo/Department of Pediatrics
800-674-6300

PENNSYLVANIA

Pregnancy Healthline/Pennsylvania Hospital (Philadelphia)
215-829-5437

Department of Reproductive Genetics/Magee-Women's Hospital (Pittsburgh)
412-647-4168

Pregnancy Safety Hotline/Western Pennsylvania Hospital (Pittsburgh)
412-687-SAFE

TEXAS

Genetic Screening and Counseling Service/Texas State Department of Mental Health and Mental Retardation (Denton)
817-383-3561

TENNESSEE

Genetics Services/Erlanger Medical Center/University of Tennessee (Chattanooga)
615-778-6112

UTAH

Pregnancy Riskline/Utah State Department of Health (Salt Lake City)
800-822-BABY (Utah, excluding Salt Lake City)
800-583-2229 (Salt Lake City area)

VERMONT

Pregnancy Risk Information Service/ University of Vermont (Burlington)
800-531-9800, 802-658-4310

WASHINGTON

Poison Control Network (Seattle)
800-732-6985, 206-526-2121

University of Washington (Seattle)
206-543-3373

WISCONSIN

Teratogen Project/University of Wisconsin (Madison)
800-442-6692, 608-262-4719

Genetics and Birth Defects Center Children's Hospital of Wisconsin (Milwaukee)
414-266-2988

Eastern Wisconsin Teratogen Service/ Genetics Section/University of Wisconsin Medical School (Milwaukee)
414-283-6029

CANADA

Motherisk/Division of Clinical
 Pharmacology/Hospital for Sick
 Children (Toronto, Ontario)
416-598-6780
 They will answer anyone's questions
about the effects of chemicals, radiation, or drugs on pregnancy.

Safe-Start Program/Chedoke-
 McMaster Hospitals (Hamilton,
 Ontario)
416-521-2100, extension 6788

Ottawa Motherisk/Children's Hospital
 of Eastern Ontario (Ottawa,
 Ontario)
613-737-2320

FRAME Program/Children's Hospital
 of Western Ontario (London,
 Ontario)
519-685-8140

Department of Medical Genetics/
 University of British Columbia/
 University Hospital (Vancouver,
 B.C.)
604-875-2157 (Shaughnessy site)

ASSOCIATIONS

The *Guide to Selected National Genetic
Voluntary Organizations* is available
from the National Center for Education in Maternal and Child Health,
38th and R Streets, N.W., Washington, D.C. 20057 (202-625-8400).
NCEMCH is a source of publications
and research information on genetic
conditions, breast-feeding, and numerous other infant or maternal health
issues. The following are a selected

number of other organizations providing information and referrals regarding
the prevention of birth defects:

Association of Birth Defect Children, Betty Mekdeci, 5400 Diplomat
Circle, Apartment 270, Orlando, Fla.
32810 (407-629-1466). This is a nonprofit clearinghouse for information
about birth defects. Mekdeci publishes
a quarterly newsletter, refers families to
resources and to other families with
similar conditions, and collects data
about birth defect causes and prevention.

March of Dimes Birth Defects
Foundation, 1275 Mamaroneck Avenue, White Plains, N.Y. 10605
(914-428-7100). This is a not-for-
profit voluntary health agency that provides grants for research, organizes
fund-raising, and supports community
programs to educate Americans about
all birth defects.

MUMS—Mothers United for Moral
Support, Julie Gordon, 150 Custer
Court, Green Bay, Wis. 54301
(414-336-5333). This is a self-help
group for parents or foster parents of a
child with any disability; it links families dealing with the same problems;
includes 260 different disabilities.

Muscular Dystrophy Association,
3561 East Sunrise Drive, Tucson, Ariz.
85718 (602-529-2000).

National Down Syndrome Society,
666 Broadway, New York, N.Y. 10012
(800-221-4602, 212-460-9330).

National Network to Prevent Birth
Defects, Box 15309, Southeast Station, Washington, D.C. 20003
(202-543-5450). Coordinator Erik
Jansson collects data, lobbies govern-

ment, and publishes a ten-page newsletter ($10 membership fee).

National Organization for Rare Disorders, P.O. Box 8925, New Fairfield, Conn. 06812 (203-746-6518).

The Arc (formerly the Association for Retarded Citizens), P.O. Box 300649, Arlington, Tex. 76010 (817-261-6003). Some of ARC's 1300 chapters focus on adults, some children, and some both.

United Cerebral Palsy Association-National, 7 Penn Plaza, New York, N.Y. 10001 (800-872-1827, 212-268-6655).

RESOURCES FOR A SAFE HOME ENVIRONMENT

Alternatives, a fact sheet from the Washington Toxics Coalition. The coalition has created fourteen of these excellently researched four-page guides to prevention and control of pests, heavy metal contamination, and other environmental pollutants. ($1 each or a set of fourteen for $8.) Washington Toxics Coalition, 4516 University Way NE, Seattle, Wash. 98105 (206-632-1545).

Safe Home Digest, a sixteen-page monthly newsletter on products, book reviews, home test kits, and environmental issues related to healthy homes. It costs $27.96 per year, payable to Lloyd Publishing Inc., 24 East Avenue, Apartment 1300, New Canaan, Conn. 06840 (203-966-2099).

Greenkeeping, a twelve-page bimonthly newsletter on nontoxic and environmentally safe products and procedures related to home life. It costs

$22.50 per year and is available from Box 110, Annandale-on-Hudson, N.Y. 12504 (914-246-6948).

BOOKS

REFERENCE

The Family Genetic Sourcebook, by Benjamin A. Pierce (John Wiley & Sons 1990), translates medical language and concepts into easily understood prose regarding inheritance, risk assessment, and how to chart your own family genetic history.

Better Health Through Natural Healing, by Dr. Ross Trattler (McGraw-Hill 1988). Subtitled "How to Get Well Without Drugs or Surgery," Trattler's book is my all-around favorite medical encyclopedia. In an affordable paperback, he thoroughly covers 107 common medical conditions from acne to yeast infections.

Healing Yourself During Pregnancy, by Joy Gardner (Crossing Press 1987). A short paperback that offers a variety of gentle, easily accomplished nontoxic, nonpharmaceutical healing techniques for common conditions.

PREGNANCY AND BIRTH

An Easier Childbirth, by Gayle Peterson, Ph.D. (Tarcher 1991). Subtitled "A Mother's Workbook for Health and Emotional Well-Being during Pregnancy and Delivery," Peterson's book focuses on the personal reality of the pregnant couple.

Having Your Baby When Others Say

No!, by Madeline P. Nugent (Avery 1991), includes how to deal with a pregnancy and the people affecting it when—because of known genetic tendencies or prenatal testing—others pressure you either to avoid pregnancy or to have an abortion.

A Good Birth, A Safe Birth, by Diana Korte and Roberta Scaer (Bantam 1990), gives you straight answers about your options for the birth experience, how to interact most advantageously with doctors and nurses, how to avoid a cesarean and if you have one, how to make it a joyful birth experience, and even how to most effectively make changes that will benefit mothers for years to come.

Birth Trap, by Yvonne Brackbill, Ph.D., June Rice, J.D., and Diony Young (Warner 1984), is a short paperback powerhouse that explains in detail high-tech procedures commonly used in hospital births and how to extricate yourself from their use, including straight talk on the consumer's bill of rights.

Alternative Birth, by Carl Jones (Tarcher 1991), discusses the many ways you can have a baby outside the conventional setting, such as having a midwife, using a childbearing center, home delivery, or requesting an in-hospital alternative birthing room. The focus is how to have a safe and successful birth experience.

Glossary

anomaly Same as malformation. A structural defect.

autosome A chromosome that is not a sex chromosome.

chromosome A structure within the nucleus of every cell, formed of a strand of deoxyribonucleic acid (DNA), which transmits genetic information. In humans, there are normally 22 pairs (44) of autosomes and 2 sex chromosomes (XX or XY), for a total of 46 chromosomes.

congenital Present at birth.

deformity A properly formed structure that is subsequently altered abnormally due to injury, disease, or disuse. May occur during gestation or after birth.

dominant A trait is dominant if only one copy of the gene determining it is needed for its expression.

embryo Unborn child from conception through eight weeks gestation.

fetus Unborn child from nine weeks gestation to birth.

gene A unit of heredity, located at a particular site along the deoxyribonucleic acid (DNA) strand that forms a chromosome. Many thousands of genes make up each chromosome, and by directing the synthesis of proteins and enzymes, they control the specific physical, physiological, and functional traits of the organism.

gestation Life in the womb, from conception to birth.

mutagen An agent causing permanent genetic change.

mutation An alteration in the genetic makeup that can be inherited.

neonatal Time period from birth through twenty-eight days of age. Neonatal is a synonym for newborn.

perinatal Time period from some time mid-pregnancy to some time in the week or weeks after birth. Exact dates vary between experts. One source suggests the twenty-eighth week of pregnancy to the end of the first week after birth.

placenta   The specialized organ that forms within a woman's uterus during pregnancy, bringing the growing fetus oxygen and nutrients from the mother's bloodstream and removing fetal-waste products. The placenta secretes hormones needed during pregnancy and is expelled as the afterbirth soon after the baby is born.

preconception   The days, months, or years before pregnancy begins.

recessive   A gene donated by one parent that does not express itself in the body of the child unless matched by a similar gene donated by the other parent.

sex chromosome   The X or Y chromosomes, which determine gender.

somatic   Pertaining to the body.

syndrome   A pattern of signs and symptoms that regularly occur together and characterize a particular abnormality.

teratogen   An agent acting upon an embryo or fetus that causes structural, functional, or developmental abnormalities that are not genetic and will not be inherited.

trisomy   The presence of one extra chromosome, so that a person's total chromosomes number 47 instead of 46.

womb   The uterus.

Select Bibliography

INTRODUCTION

Burton, Barbara K. et al. "Limb Anomalies Associated With Chorionic Villus Sampling." *Obstetrics & Gynecology* 79, no. 5 (May 1992) Part 1:726.

Jongbloet, P. H. *Mental and Physical Handicaps in Connection with Overripeness, Ovopathy.* Leiden: H. E. Stenfert Kroese N.V. (1971), pp. 10, 14, 48.

Kelley-Buchanan, Christine. *Peace of Mind During Pregnancy.* New York: Facts on File Publications, 1988.

Suchy, Sharon F., Ph.D., and Maria T. Yeager, B.S. "Down Syndrome Screening in Women under 35 with Maternal Serum hCG." *Obstetrics & Gynecology* 76, no. 1 (July 1990): 20.

Part I: *Before Pregnancy*

PRECONCEPTION CARE

Barnes, Belinda et al. "Nutrition and Pre-Conception Care (Letter)." *Lancet* (Dec. 7, 1985): 1297.

Chez, Ronald A., M.D., moderator. "Symposium: Why It's Important to Help Patients Prepare for Pregnancy." *Contemporary OB/GYN* 33, no. 6 (June 1989): 2.

Gordus, A. A. et al. "Human Hair as an Indicator of Trace Metal Environmental Exposure." *Proceedings of the First Annual NSF Trace Contaminants Conference.* (Oak Ridge, Tennessee: Oak Ridge National Laboratory (Aug. 8–10, 1973): 463.

Moos, Merry K., F.N.P., M.P.H., and Robert C. Cefalo, M.D., Ph.D. "Preconceptional Health Promotion: A Focus for Obstetric Care." *American Journal of Perinatology* 4, no. 1 (January 1987): 63.

PRE-EXISTING MEDICAL CONDITIONS

AIDS

Oxtoby, Margaret J., M.D. "Human Immunodeficiency Virus and Other Viruses in Human Milk: Placing the Issues in Broader Perspective." *Pediatric Infectious Disease* 7, no. 12 (December 1988): 825.

Rogers, Martha F., M.D. "AIDS in Children: A Review of the Clinical,

Epidemiologic and Public Health Aspects." *Pediatric Infectious Disease* 4, no. 3 (May 1985): 230.

Diabetes

Damm, Peter, M.D., and Lars Molsted-Pedersen, M.D., Ph.D. "Significant Decrease in Congenital Malformations in Newborn Infants of an Unselected Population of Diabetic Women." *American Journal of Obstetrics and Gynecology* 161, no. 5 (November 1989): 1163.

Kitzmiller, John L., M.D., et al. "Preconception Care of Diabetes: Glycemic Control Prevents Congenital Anomalies." *Journal of the American Medical Association* 265, no. 6 (Feb. 13, 1991): 731.

Krolewski, Andrzej S., M.D., Ph.D., James H. Warram, M.D., et al. "Epidemiologic Approach to the Etiology of Type 1 Diabetes Mellitus and Its Complications." *The New England Journal of Medicine* 317, no. 22 (Nov. 26, 1987): 1390.

"Perinatal Mortality and Congenital Malformations in Infants Born to Women with Insulin-Dependent Diabetes Mellitus—United States, Canada, and Europe, 1940–1988." *Morbidity and Mortality Weekly Report* (Atlanta, Ga.: Centers for Disease Control) 39, no. 21 (June 1, 1990): 363.

Epilepsy

The Epilepsy Foundation of America, 4351 Garden City Drive, Landover, Md. 20785, 800-EFA-1000. Ann Scherer, Director of Information and Education.

Occupational Hazards for Women

Baird, Donna Day, Ph.D., and Allen J. Wilcox, M.D., Ph.D. "Effects of Occupational Exposures on the Fertility of Couples. Reproductive Problems in the Workplace." Edited by Zena A. Stein and Maureen C. Hatch, Ph.D. *Occupational Medicine.* Philadelphia, Pa.: Hanley & Belfus, 1, no. 3 (July–September 1986): 361.

Barlow, Susan M., and Frank M. Sullivan. *Reproductive Hazards of Industrial Chemicals.* San Diego, Calif.: Academic Press, 1982.

Bjerkendal, Tor. "Occupation and Outcome of Pregnancy: A Population-Based Study in Norway." In *Prevention of Physical and Mental Congenital Defects, Part B,* edited by Maurice Marois. New York: Alan R. Liss, 1985.

Erickson, J. David. "Birth Defects and Parental Occupation." In *Pregnant Women at Work,* edited by Geoffrey Chamberlain. London: Royal Society of Medicine, and London: Macmillan Press, 1984.

Gabbe, Steven G. "Reproductive Hazards of the American Life Style." In *Pregnant Women at Work,* p. 57.

Haas, Joanna F., M.D., and David Schottenfeld, M.D. "Risks to the Offspring from Parental Occupational Exposures." *Journal of Occupational Medicine* 21, no. 9 (September 1979): 607.

Kline, Jennie K., Ph.D. "Maternal Occupation: Effects on Spontaneous Abortions and Malformations; Reproductive Problems in the Workplace." *Occupational Medicine* 1, no. 3 (July–September 1986): 381.

Mattison, Donald R. "What Evidence Is Required to Identify a Chemical as a Reproductive Hazard?" In *Pregnant Women at Work*, p. 157.

Paul, Maureen, M.D., and Jay Himmelstein, M.D. "Reproductive Hazards in the Workplace: What the Practitioner Needs to Know About Chemical Exposures." *Obstetrics & Gynecology* 71, no. 6, Part 1 (June 1988): 921.

Peters, John M. et al. "Brain Tumors in Children and Occupational Exposure of Parents." *Science* 213 (July 10, 1981): 235.

Savitz, David A. et al. "Self-Reported Exposure to Pesticides and Radiation Related to Pregnancy Outcome." *Public Health Reports*, 104, no. 5 (September/October 1989): 473.

Schwartz, David A., M.D., and James P. LoGerfo, M.D. "Congenital Limb Reduction Defects in the Agricultural Setting." *American Journal of Public Health* 78, no. 6 (June 1988): 656.

Tikkanen, Jorma, and Olli P. Heinonen. "Cardiovascular Malformations and Organic Solvent Exposure During Pregnancy in Finland." *American Journal of Industrial Medicine* 14 (1988): 1.

THE FATHER'S ROLE

Abel, Ernest L. et al. "The Effects of Early Marijuana Exposure." *Handbook of Behavioral Teratology*. Edited by Edward P. Riley and Charles V. Vorhees. New York: Plenum Press, 1986.

Aschengrau, Ann, Sc.D., and Richard R. Monson, M.D., Sc.D. "Paternal Military Service in Vietnam and the Risk of Late Adverse Pregnancy Outcome." *American Journal of Public Health* 80, no. 10 (October 1990): 1218.

Buckley, Jonathan D. et al. "Occupational Exposures of Parents of Children with Acute Nonlymphocytic Leukemia: A Report from the Childrens Cancer Study Group." *Cancer Research* 49 (July 15, 1989): 4030.

Friedman, J. M., M.D., Ph.D. "Genetic Disease in the Offspring of Older Fathers." *Obstetrics & Gynecology* 57, no. 6 (June 1981): 745.

Haas, Joanna F., M.D., and David Schottenfeld, M.D. "Risks to the Offspring from Parental Occupational Exposures." *Journal of Occupational Medicine* 21, no. 9 (September 1979): 607.

Little, Ruth E., and Charles F. Sing. "Father's Drinking and Infant Birth Weight: Report of an Association." *Teratology* 36 (August 1987): 59.

Lowengart, Ruth A. et al. "Childhood Leukemia and Parents' Occupational and Home Exposures." *Journal of the National Cancer Institute* 79, no. 1 (July 1987): 39.

Olshan, Andrew F. et al. "Birth Defects Among Offspring of Firemen." *American Journal of Epidemiology* 131, no. 2 (February 1990): 312.

Olshan, Andrew F. et al. "Paternal Occupational Exposures and the Risk of Down Syndrome." *American Journal of Human Genetics* 44 (May 1989): 646.

Peters, John M. et al. "Brain Tumors in Children and Occupational Exposure of Parents." *Science* 213 (July 10, 1981): 235.

Savitz, David A., Ph.D., et al. "Self-Reported Exposure to Pesticides and Radiation Related to Pregnancy Outcome—Results from National Natality and Fetal Mortality Surveys." *Public Health Reports* 104, no. 5 (September–October 1989): 473.

Soyka, Lester F., M.D., and Justin M. Joffee, Ph.D. "Male Mediated Effects on Offspring." *Drug and Chemical Risks to the Fetus and Newborn.* Edited by Richard H. Schwarz, M.D., and Sumner J. Yaffe, M.D. New York: Alan R. Liss, 1980.

Vaishwanar, P. S., and B. V. Deshkar. "Ascorbic Acid Content and Quality of Human Semen." *American Journal of Obstetrics and Gynecology* 95, no. 8 (August 1966): 1080.

Part II: *During Pregnancy*

PRENATAL CARE

Institute of Medicine, Committee on Nutritional Status During Pregnancy and Lactation of the Food and Nutrition Board. *Nutrition During Pregnancy: Weight Gain, Nutrient Supplements.* Washington, D.C.: National Academy Press, 1990.

Jansson, Erik. "Components of a National Program to Reduce Birth Defects, Learning Disability, Very Low Birth Weight, and Child Abuse Rates by 50 Percent and Childhood Cancer by 30 Percent." *National Network to Prevent Birth Defects Position Paper* (Oct. 21, 1987, updated to 1990).

Olds, David L., Ph.D., et al. "Improving the Delivery of Prenatal Care and Outcomes of Pregnancy: A Randomized Trial of Nurse Home Visitation." *Pediatrics* 77, no. 1 (January 1986): 16.

Orstead, Catherine, M.S., R.D., et al. "Efficacy of Prenatal Nutrition Counseling: Weight Gain, Infant Birth Weight, and Cost-Effectiveness." *Journal of the American Dietetic Association* 85, no. 1 (January 1985): 40.

Papiernik, Emile, M.D. et al., eds. "Effective Prevention of Preterm Birth: The French Experience Measured at Haguenau." *Birth Defects: Original Article Series* 25, no. 1. White Plains, N.Y.: March of Dimes Birth Defects Foundation, 1989: 107.

PREMATURITY, LOW BIRTH WEIGHT, AND STRESS

Binsacca, Donald B., M.S., et al. "Factors Associated with Low Birthweight in an Inner-City Population: The Role of Financial Problems." *American Journal of Public Health* 77, no. 4 (April 1987): 505.

Homer, C. J., S. A. James, and E. Siegel. "Work-Related Psychosocial Stress and Risk of Preterm, Low Birthweight Delivery." *American Journal of Public Health* 80, no. 2 (February 1990): 173.

McAnarney, Elizabeth R., M.D., and Catherine Stevens-Simon, M.D. "Maternal Psychological Stress/Depression and Low Birth Weight: Is There a Relationship?" *American Journal of Disease in Children* 144 (July 1990): 789.

Mehl, Lewis E., M.D., Ph.D. "Preventing Prematurity." *Mothering* 49 (Fall 1988): 70.

Meis, Paul J., M.D., et al. "Regional Program for Prevention of Premature Birth in North Carolina." *American Journal of Obstetrics and Gynecology* 157, no. 3 (September 1987): 550.

Omer, Haim. "A Hypnotic Relaxation Technique for the Treatment of Premature Labor." *American Journal of Clinical Hypnosis* 29, no. 3 (January 1987): 206.

Omer, Haim, Ph.D., and George S. Everly, Jr., Ph.D. "Psychological Factors in Preterm Labor: Critical Review and Theoretical Synthesis." *American Journal of Psychiatry* 145, no. 12 (December 1988): 1507.

Papiernik, Emile, M.D. "Preventing Prematurity" (Letter to the Editor). *Journal of the American Medical Association* 262, no. 22 (Dec. 8, 1989): 3128.

Scialli, Anthony R. "Is Stress a Developmental Toxin?" *Reproductive Toxicology* 1, no. 3 (1987/1988): 163.

Williamson, H. A., Jr., M. LeFevre, and M. Hector, Jr. "Association Between Life Stress and Serious Perinatal Complications." *Journal of Family Practice* 29, no. 5 (November 1989): 489.

Zuckerman, Barry, M.D., et al. "Depressive Symptoms During Pregnancy: Relationship to Poor Health Behaviors." *American Journal of Obstetrics and Gynecology* 160 (May 1989): 110.

DIET AND NUTRITION

Hurley, Lucille. "Trace Elements and Their Interactions as Causes of Congenital Defects." Workshop on Nutrition, International Conference of the Institut de la Vie, Strausbourg, France; 10/10–17/82. In *Prevention of Physical and Mental Congenital Defects, Part B: Epidemiology, Early Detection and Therapy, and Environmental Factors.* New York: Alan R. Liss, 1985.

Institute of Medicine, National Academy of Sciences, Subcommittee on Nutritional Status and Weight Gain During Pregnancy. *Nutrition During Pregnancy.* Washington, D.C.: National Academy Press, 1990.

Klingberg, Marcus A. et al. "The Etiology of Central Nervous System Defects." *Neurobehavioral Teratology.* Amsterdam, The Netherlands: Elsevier Science Publishers, 1984.

Mulinare, Joseph et al. "Periconceptional Use of Multivitamins and the Occurrence of Neural Tube Defects." *Journal of the American Medical Association* 260, no. 21 (Dec. 2, 1988): 3141.

Peer, L. A. et al. "Effect of Vitamins on Human Teratology." *Plastic and Reconstructive Surgery* 34, no. 4 (October 1964): 358.

Tolarova, M. "Periconceptional Supplementation with Vitamins and Folic Acid to Prevent Recurrence of Cleft Lip." *Lancet* 2:8291 (July 24, 1982): 217.

Walford, Roy L., M.D. "Selenium Content of Various Foods." In *The 120 Year Diet.* New York: Pocket Books, 1986.

Yates, J., M. Ferguson-Smith, A. Shenkin et al. "Vitamin Status and Neural Tube Defects." *Journal of Medical Genetics* 22 (October 1985): 394.

PRESCRIPTION AND OVER-THE-COUNTER DRUGS

Brackbill, Yvonne, M.D. (quoted in Editorial). *Birth and the Family Journal* 5, no. 2 (Summer 1978): 56.

Bracken, Michael, and Theodore Holford. "Exposure to Prescribed Drugs in Pregnancy and Association with Congenital Malformations." *Obstetrics & Gynecology* 58, no. 3 (September 1981): 336.

Brent, Robert L. Table 2: Relative Contributions of Various Causes to the Frequency of Human Malformations. In "The Complexities of Solving the Problem of Human Malformations." In *Teratogen Update: Environmentally Induced Birth Defect Risks.* New York: Alan R. Liss, 1986.

Brown, Roger M., and Rachelle H. B. Fishman. "An Overview and Summary of the Behavioral and Neural Consequences of Perinatal Exposure to Psychotropic Drugs." In *Neurobehavioral Teratology.* Amsterdam, The Netherlands: Elsevier Science Publishers, 1984.

Council on Scientific Affairs. "Effects of Toxic Chemicals on the Reproductive System." *Journal of the American Medical Association* 253, no. 23 (June 21, 1985: 3431.

Farwell, Jacquelin R. et al. "Phenobarbital for Febrile Seizures—Effects on Intelligence and on Seizure Recurrence." *New England Journal of Medicine* 322, no. 6 (Feb. 8, 1990): 364.

Goldman, Allen S., M.D. "Critical Periods of Prenatal Toxic Insults." In *Drug and Chemical Risks to the Fetus and Newborn.* Edited by Richard H. Schwarz, M.D. and Sumner J. Yaffe, M.D. New York: Alan R. Liss, 1980.

Laegreid, Liv et al. "Teratogenic Effects of Benzodiazepine Use During Pregnancy." *Journal of Pediatrics* 114 (January 1989): 126.

London, Robert S. "Saccharin and Aspartame: Are They Safe to Consume During Pregnancy?" *The Journal of Reproductive Medicine* 33, no. 1 (January 1988): 17.

U.S. Dept. of Health and Human Services, Immunization Practices Advisory Committee (ACIP). "Use of Immunobiologics in Pregnancy." *U.S. Pharmacist* (February 1985): 66.

Vanoverloop, D. et al. "Effects of Anticonvulsants on Intelligence Function at Ages 4 to 8 Years." Behavioral Teratology Society Abstracts. *Teratology* 37, no. 5 (May 1988): 520.

Webb, James L., Ph.D. "Nutritional Effects of Oral Contraceptive Use: A Review." *Journal of Reproductive Medicine* 25, no. 4 (October 1980): 150.

Zhu, Ming-xia, and Shu-shun Zhou. "Reduction of the Teratogenic Effects of Phenytoin by Folic Acid and a Mixture of Folic Acid, Vitamins, and Amino Acids: A Preliminary Trial." *Epilepsia* 30, no. 2 (Mar.-Apr. 1989): 246.

RECREATIONAL DRUGS

Alcohol

Mills, James L. et al. "Maternal Alcohol Consumption and Birth Weight." *Journal of the American Medical Association* 252:14 (October 12, 1984): 1875.

Warren, Kenneth R., Ph.D., and Richard J. Bast. "Alcohol-related Birth Defects: An Update." *Public Health Reports* 103, no. 6 (Nov.-Dec. 1988): 638.

Coffee and Tea

Bershoff, Stanley, Ph.D. "Measure Your Caffeine Intake." In *The Tufts University Guide to Total Nutrition*. New York: HarperCollins, 1991.

Pieters, J. J. L. "Nutritional Teratogens." In *Prevention of Physical and Mental Defects, Part B: Epidemiology, Early Detection and Therapy, and Environmental Factors*. New York: Alan R. Liss, 1985.

Srisuphan, W., and M. Bracken. "Caffeine Consumption During Pregnancy and Association with Late Spontaneous Abortion." *American Journal of Obstetrics and Gynecology* 154 (January 1986): 14.

U.S. Department of Health and Human Services, Food and Drug Administration. *Caffeine and Pregnancy*. HHS Publication No. (FDA) 81–1081.

Marijuana and Heroin

Abel, Ernest L. et al. "The Effects of Early Marijuana Exposure." In *Handbook of Behavioral Teratology*. Edited by Edward P. Riley and Charles V. Vorhees. New York: Plenum Press, 1986.

Fried, Peter A. "Prenatal and Postnatal Consequences of Marihuana [sic] Use During Pregnancy." *Neurobehavioral Teratology*. Amsterdam, The Netherlands: Elsevier Science Publishers, 1984.

Zagon, Ian S., and Patricia J. McLaughlin. "An Overview of the Neurobehavioral Sequelae of Perinatal Opioid Exposure." *Neurobehavioral Teratology*. Amsterdam, The Netherlands: Elsevier Science Publishers, 1984.

Nicotine

Bergner, Paul. "Herbs to Aid in Nicotine Withdrawal." *Townsend Letter for Doctors* 84 (July 1990): 443.

Bracken, Michael, and Theodore Holford. "Exposure to Prescribed Drugs in Pregnancy and Congenital Malformations." *Obstetrics & Gynecology* 58, no. 3 (September 1981): 336.

Meyer, M. B., and J. A. Tonascia. "Maternal Smoking, Pregnancy Complications, and Perinatal Mortality." *American Journal of Obstetrics and Gynecology* 128, no. 5 (July 1, 1977): 494.

Preston-Martin, Susan et al. "N-Nitroso Compounds and Childhood Brain Tumors—A Case Control Study." *Cancer Research* 42 (December 1982): 5240.

Sexton, Mary et al. "Prenatal Exposure to Tobacco: Effects on Cognitive Functioning at Age Three." *International Journal of Epidemiology* 19, no. 1 (March 1990): 72.

Stjernfeldt, Michael et al. "Maternal Smoking During Pregnancy and the Risk of Childhood Cancer." *Lancet* 2:8508 (Sept. 20, 1986): 687.

ENVIRONMENTAL TOXICANTS

Air

The major sources of information for this section were interviews with the following experts from the Environmental Protection Agency: Michael Berry, Ph.D. (Deputy Director, Environmental Criteria and Assessment Office), Patty Bubar, Ph.D. (Chief, Office of Radiation Programs), Susan Conrath, Ph.D. (Measurement and Characterization Section), Michael Davis, Ph.D. (Office of Research and Development), Carole Kimmel, Ph.D. (Office of Health and Environmental Assessment), Gary Kimmel, Ph.D. (Office of Health and Environmental Assessment), Sherry Selevan, Ph.D. (Office of Health and Environmental Assessment), Chon Shoaf, Ph.D. (Chief, Hazardous Pollutant Assessment Branch), and Lance Wallace (Office of Research and Development).

Additional information was obtained from Jose Kirchner, of the American Lung Association, Sacramento chapter, and William Wolverton, of Wolverton Environmental Services, Piscayune, Miss.

Water

Bean, Judy A. et al. "Drinking Water and Cancer Incidence in Iowa." *American Journal of Epidemiology* 116, no. 6 (December 1982): 912.

Fagliano, Jerald, MPH, et al. "Drinking Water Contamination and the Incidence of Leukemia: An Ecological Study." *American Journal of Public Health* 80, no. 10 (October 1990): 1209.

Miller, Gregory D., Ph.D. "Interactions Between Lead and Essential Elements: Behavioral Consequences." *The Nutrition Report* 9, no. 2 (February 1991): 9.

Hidden Contamination

Agocs, Mary M., M.D., et al. "Mercury Exposure from Interior Latex Paint." *The New England Journal of Medicine* 323, no. 16 (Oct. 18, 1990): 1096.

Graziano, Joseph, and Conrad Blum. "Lead Exposure from Lead Crystal." *Lancet* 337 (Jan. 19, 1991): 141.

Needleman, Herbert et al. "The Relationship Between Prenatal Exposure to Lead and Congenital Anomalies." *Journal of the American Medical Association* 251, no. 22 (June 8, 1984): 2956.

Rabin, Richard, MSPH. "Warnings Unheeded: A History of Child Lead Poisoning." *American Journal of Public Health* 79, no. 12 (December 1989): 1668.

Water Exposure and Pregnancy Outcomes. Epidemiological Studies and Surveillance Section, California Department of Health Services (May 1988).

Electromagnetic Radiation

Antman, Mark, and Stewart Maurer, Ph.D. "Viewpoint: Looking at Lightboxes in a New Light." *Photo District News* 11, no. 11 (Oct. 1991): 140. For back issues of the magazine, contact *Photo District News* at (212) 677-8418, 49 E. 21st St., New York, N.Y. 10010.

Bean, Judy A. et al. "Drinking Water and Cancer Incidence in Iowa, II Radioactivity in Drinking Water." *American Journal of Epidemiology* 116, no. 6 (December 1982): 924.

Becker, Robert O., M.D. *Cross Currents.* Los Angeles: Jeremy P. Tarcher, 1990.

Brent, Robert L. "The Effect of Embryonic and Fetal Exposure to X-ray, Microwaves, and Ultrasound: Counseling the Pregnant and Nonpregnant Patient About These Risks." *Seminars in Oncology* 16, no. 5 (October 1989): 347.

Gofman, John W., M.D., Ph.D. "Radiation-Induced Cancer from Low Dose Exposure." San Francisco: Committee for Nuclear Responsibility, 1990:1.

Goldhaber, Marilyn K. et al. "The Risk of Miscarriage and Birth Defects Among Women Who Use Visual Display Terminals During Pregnancy." *American Journal of Industrial Medicine* 13, no. 6 (1988): 695.

Jankowski, Carol, R.N., M.Ed. "Radiation and Pregnancy: Putting the Risks in Proportion." *American Journal of Nursing* 86:3 (March 1986): 261.

Kneale, George V., and Alice M. Stewart. "Childhood Cancers in the U.K. and Their Relation to Background Radiation." In *Radiation and Health: The Biological Effects of Low-level Exposure to Ionizing Radiation.* Richard Southwood, Robin Russell, et al., eds. Edited proceedings of a symposium, "The Biological Effects of Radiation," held Nov. 25–26, 1986 at Hammersmith Hospital, London. London: John Wiley and Sons, 1987:203.

Savitz, David A. et al. "Case-control Study of Childhood Cancers and Exposure to 60-Hz Magnetic Fields." *American Journal of Epidemiology* 128, no. 1 (July 1988): 21.

Schnorr, Teresa M., Ph.D., et al. "Video Display Terminals and the Risk of Spontaneous Abortion." *The New England Journal of Medicine* 324, no. 11 (March 14, 1991): 727.

Tanaka, Y. et al. "Studies on Inhibition of Intestinal Absorption of Radio-Active Strontium." *Canadian Medical Association Journal* 99 (July 1968): 169.

Wertheimer, Nancy, and Ed Leeper. "Fetal Loss Associated with Two Seasonal Sources of Electromagnetic Field Exposure." *American Journal of Epidemiology* 129, no. 1 (January 1989): 220.

Pesticides

Jaffe, Russell, M.D., Ph.D. "Sixteen Million Americans Sensitive to Pesticides." *Townsend Letter for Doctors* 89 (December 1990): 869.

Kricker, Anne et al. "Women and the Environment: A Study of Congenital Limb Anomalies." *Community Health Studies* X, no. 1 (1986): 1.

Mactutus, Charles F., and Hugh A. Tilson. "Psychogenic and Neurogenic Abnormalities after Perinatal Insecticide Exposure." In *Handbook of Behavioral Teratology,* edited by E. P. Riley and C. V. Vorhees. New York: Plenum Press, 1986.

"On Pests and Pesticides." *The Human Ecologist,* no. 45 (Spring 1990): 22.

Russell-Manning, Betsy. *Malathion: Toxic Time Bomb.* San Francisco: Greensward Press, 1990.

U.S. Congress, Office of Technology Assessment. "Neurotoxicity: Identifying and Controlling Poisons of the Nervous System." OTA-BA-436. U.S. Government Printing Office, 1990.

EXERCISE

Cassidy-Brinn, Ginny, R.N. et al. *Woman-Centered Pregnancy and Childbirth.* Pittsburgh, Pa.: Cleis Press, 1984.

Clapp, James F. III, M.D. "The Effects of Maternal Exercise on Early Pregnancy Outcome." *American Journal of Obstetrics and Gynecology* 161, no. 6 (December 1989): 1453.

Samuels, Mike, M.D., and Nancy Samuels. *The Well Pregnancy Book.* New York: Summit, 1986.

GESTATIONAL DIABETES

Weiss, Peter A. M., and Donald R. Coustan. *Gestational Diabetes.* New York: Springer-Verlag, 1988.

INFECTIOUS DISEASES

Centers for Disease Control. "Sexually Transmitted Diseases Treatment Guidelines, September, 1989." *Morbidity and Mortality Weekly Report Recommendations and Reports* 38, no. S-8 (Sept. 1, 1989).

Fuccillo, David A. "Congenital Varicella." In *Teratogen Update: Environmentally Induced Birth Defect Risks,* edited by John L. Sever and Robert L. Brent. New York: Alan R. Liss, 1986.

Grossman, John H. III. "Congenital Syphilis." In *Teratogen Update,* p. 113.
———. "Preventing Neonatal Herpes Simplex Infections: An Obstetrician's Perspective." In *Prevention of Physical and Mental Congenital Defects, Part B,* edited by Maurice Marois. New York: Alan R. Liss, 1985.

Korones, Sheldon B. "Congenital Rubella—An Encapsulated Review." In *Teratogen Update,* p. 77.

Larsen, John W., Jr. "Congenital Toxoplasmosis." In *Teratogen Update,* p. 97.

Moore, Keith L., M.Sc., Ph.D., F.I.A.C. "Before We Are Born: Basic Embryology and Birth Defects." In *Congenital Malformations and Their Causes,* 3d ed. Philadelphia, Pa.: W. B. Saunders, 1989.

Nahmias, Andre J., and Mary G. Schwahn. "Neonatal Herpes Simplex: A Worldwide Disease Which Is Potentially Preventable and Treatable." In *Prevention of Physical and Mental Congenital Defects, Part B,* p. 355.

Reynolds, D. W. et al. "Congenital Cytomegalovirus Infections." In *Teratogen Update,* p. 93.

LABOR AND DELIVERY

Brackbill, Yvonne. "Presentation." *Birth and the Family Journal* 5:2 (Summer 1978): 55.

Bracken, Michael, and Theodore Holford. "Exposure to Prescribed Drugs in Pregnancy and Congenital Malformations." *Obstetrics & Gynecology* 58, no. 3 (September 1981): 336.

Coletti, L. "Relationship between Pregnancy and Birth Complications and the Later Development of Learning Disability." *Journal of Learning Disabilities* 12 (December 1979): 659.

Cooperative Research Group of Moxibustion Version. "Studies on Correcting Abnormal Fetal Positions by Moxibustion to Zhiyin Points." In *Advances in Acupuncture and Acupuncture Anaesthesia* (abstracts of papers presented at the National Symposium of Acupuncture, Moxibustion and Acupuncture Anaesthesia, Beijing, June 1–5, 1979). Beijing, China: The People's Medical Publishing House, 1980.

Croughan-Minihane, MS, et al. "Morbidity Among Breech Infants According to Method of Delivery." *Obstetrics & Gynecology* 75, no. 5 (May 1990): 821.

Frager, Neal B., M.D., and Fred S. Miyazaki, M.D. "Intrauterine Monitoring of Contractions During Breast Stimulation." *Obstetrics & Gynecology* 69, no. 5 (May 1987): 767.

Freeman, Robert, M.D. "Intrapartum Fetal Monitoring—A Disappointing Story." *The New England Journal of Medicine* 322:9 (March 1, 1990): 624.

Gabbe, S. et al. "Umbilical Cord Compression Associated with Amniotomy: Laboratory Observations." *American Journal of Obstetrics and Gynecology* 126 (October 1976): 353.

Inlander, Charles B., Lowell S. Levin, and Ed Weiner. "The Blues of the Birth." *Medicine On Trial*. New York: Prentice-Hall Press, 1988.

Jansson, Erik. "Components of a National Program to Reduce Birth Defects, Learning Disability, Very Low Birth Weight, and Child Abuse Rates by 50 Percent and Childhood Cancer by 30 Percent." *National Network to Prevent Birth Defects* (October 21, 1987 updated to 1990): 50.

Luthy, David A., M.D., Kirwood K. Shy, M.D., M.P.H. et al. "A Randomized Trial of Electronic Fetal Monitoring in Preterm Labor." *Obstetrics & Gynecology* 69, no. 5 (May 1987): 687.

Mazze, Richard I., M.D., and Bengt Kallen, M.D., Ph.D. "Reproductive Outcome After Anesthesia and Operation During Pregnancy: A Registry Study of 5405 Cases." *American Journal of Obstetrics and Gynecology* 161, no. 5 (November 1989): 1178.

Myers, Stephen A., and Norbert Gleicher. "A Successful Program to Lower Cesarean-Section Rates." *New England Journal of Medicine* 319, no. 23 (Dec. 8, 1988): 1511.

Ralston, David H., M.D., and Sol M. Shnider, M.D. "The Fetal and Neonatal Effects of Regional Anesthesia in Obstetrics." *Anesthesiology* 48 (Jan.-June 1978): 34.

Shy, Kirkwood K., M.D., M.P.H., et al. "Effects of Electronic Fetal-Heart-Rate Monitoring, as Compared with Periodic Auscultation, on the Neurologic Development of Premature Infants." *New England Journal of Medicine* 322, no. 9 (March 1, 1990): 588.

Studd, J. W. W. et al. "The Effect of Lumbar Epidural Analgesia on the Rate of Cervical Dilatation and the Outcome of Labour of Spontaneous Onset." *British Journal of Obstetrics and Gynaecology* 87 (November 1980): 1015.

Part III: *After Pregnancy*

INFANT FEEDING

American Academy of Pediatrics Committee on Drugs. "Transfer of Drugs and Other Chemicals Into Human Milk." *Pediatrics* 84, no. 5 (November 1989): 924.

Berlin, Cheston M., Jr. "The Excretion of Drugs in Human Milk." In *Drug and Chemical Risks to the Fetus and Newborn*, edited by Richard H. Schwarz, M.D., and Sumner J. Yaffe, M.D. New York: Alan R. Liss, 1980.

"Extensive Study Underscores Benefits of Breastfeeding; Good Nutrition During Lactation." *News from the Institute of Medicine* (Feb. 19, 1991).

Mofenson, Howard C., M.D., and Thomas R. Caraccio, Pharm.D. "Drugs, Breast Milk, and Infants." *Pediatric Therapeutics & Toxicology/ Supplement* (March 1988): S1.

Moses, Lenette S. "Drugs and Breastmilk." *Mothering* 56 (Summer 1990): 68.

Neifert, Marianne R., M.D., and Joy M. Seacat, CHA, MS. "A Guide to Successful Breast-feeding." *Contemporary Pediatrics* 3 (July 1986): 1.

Rayburn, William F., M.D., and Frederick P. Zuspan, M.D., eds. *Drug Therapy in Obstetrics and Gynecology.* Old Tappan, N.J.: Appleton-Century-Crofts (Prentice-Hall), 1986.

SUDDEN INFANT DEATH SYNDROME

Centers for Disease Control. "Seasonality in Sudden Infant Death Syndrome." *Morbidity and Mortality Weekly Report* 39, no. 49 (Dec. 14, 1990): 891.

De Jonge, Guus A., and Adele C. Engelberts. "Cot Deaths and Sleeping Position." *Lancet* II, no. 8672 (November 11, 1989): 1149.

Hoffman, H. J. et al. "Risk Factors For SIDS: Results of the National Institute of Child Health and Human Development SIDS Cooperative Epidemiological Study." *Annals of the New York Academy of Science* 533 (August 1988): 13.

Sears, William, M.D. "Nighttime Parenting and Sudden Infant Death Syndrome." *Nighttime Parenting: How to Get Your Baby and Child to Sleep.* New York: Penguin Books, 1985.

Wigfield, Ruth E. et al. "Can the Fall in Avon's Sudden Infant Death Rate be Explained by Changes in Sleeping Position?" *British Medical Journal* 304, no. 6822 (February 1, 1992): 282.

YOUR CHILD'S ENVIRONMENT

Amitai, Yona et al. "Hazards of 'Deleading' Homes of Children with Lead Poisoning." *American Journal of Diseases of Children* 141 (July 1987).

Farfel, Mark R., Sc.D., and J. Julian Chisolm Jr., M.D. "Health and Environmental Outcomes of Traditional and Modified Practices for Abatement of Residential Lead-Based Paint." *American Journal of Public Health* 80, no. 10 (October 1990): 1240.

Henshaw, Denis L. et al. "Radon as a Causative Factor in Induction of Myeloid Leukaemia and Other Cancers." *Lancet* 335, no. 8696 (April 28, 1990): 1008.

Moon, Charles et al. "Main and Interaction Effects of Metallic Pollutants on Cognitive Functioning." *Journal of Learning Disabilities* 18, no. 4 (April 1985): 217.

Needleman, Herbert L. "The Long-Term Effects of Exposure to Low Doses of Lead in Childhood." *New England Journal of Medicine* 322, no. 2 (Jan. 11, 1990): 83.

O'Brien, Mary. "Are Pesticides Taking Away the Ability of Our Children to Learn?" *Journal of Pesticide Reform* 10, no. 4 (Winter 1990–91): 4.

Stewart, A., and G. V. Kneale. "Radiation Dose Effects in Relation to Obstetric X-rays and Childhood Cancers." *Lancet* 1, no. 7658 (June 6, 1970): 1185.

Index

Abdul-Karim, Raja W., 72
Accutane, 66, 69
Acetaminophen, 70–71
Achondroplasia, 9, 39
Acne medications, 69
Acupuncture, 76–77, 80. *See also*
    Moxibustion
Advil, 71
Afro-Americans, 4, 11
    and Sudden Infant Death
        Syndrome, 141
Age, maternal, 15–16
    and Down syndrome, 15–16
Age, paternal, 15–16, 39
    and Down syndrome, 15–16
Agent Orange, 43–44, 45
Agriculture, 148
AIDS (Acquired Immune Deficiency
        Syndrome), 27–28
Air pollution, 83–87
    indoor, 84–87
    outdoor, 83–84
Albinism, 11
Alcohol consumption, 5, 14, 25, 52,
        75–77, 152
    breast-feeding and, 134
    checklist, 76–77
    risks, 75–76
    sperm and, 41
Alcoholics Anonymous, 76
Allergies, 12
Alpha-fetoprotein (AFP), 17
Alternative Birth (Jones), 165
Aluminum, 145
American Academy of Pediatrics, 136
American College of Obstetricians and
        Gynecologists (ACOG), 122–123
    on vaginal birth after cesarean, 125

"American College of Obstetrics and
        Gynecology Pregnancy Exercise
        Program" (videotape), 103
American Diabetes Association, 32
American Dietetic Association, 62
American Holistic Medical
        Association, 62
American Self-Help Clearinghouse, 56
Aminopterin, 66, 68
Aminotriptyline, 68
Amniocentesis, 18–19
Amphetamine, and breast-feeding
        and, 134
Anaprox, 69
Anemia, hemolytic, 68
Anemia, sickle-cell, 9, 11, 158
    blood test for, 11, 17
    ethnic group and, 10
    frequency of occurrence, 3, 158
Anencephaly, 153
    frequency of occurrence, 153
    MSAFP testing for, 17
    ultrasound testing for, 18
    vitamin supplements and, 58–59
Anesthetics during labor, 123–124
    long-range effects of, 123–24, 127
Antibiotics, 42, 68
    and breast-feeding, 134
Anticancer drugs, 42, 66, 67, 68
    and breast-feeding, 134
Anticonvulsant medications, 41, 42,
        66, 69
    and birth defects, 32
    breast-feeding and, 134
    and folic acid, 62
Antidepressants, 68
Antiepileptic drugs, 69
Antihistamines, and breast-feeding, 134

Anti-inflammatory medications, 69
Anxiety. *See* Stress, emotional
Arsenic, 145
Artemis Speaks (Koehler), 128
Ashford, Nicholas A., 87
Asians, 4
Aspartame, 71
Aspirin, 60, 67, 70–71
    and breast-feeding, 135–36
Association for Retarded Citizens, 4
Associations, 163–64
Attitude, 53, 55
Auscultation, 121–22
Automobile exhaust fumes, 43

Bactrim, 68
Baer, Linda, 89
Becker, Robert O., 98
Beckwith, Bruce, 14
Bed, placement of, 97
Before Pregnancy Health Inventory, 25
Bendroflumethiazide, and breast-feeding
    and, 134
Benzene compounds, 42
Benzodiazepines, during labor/
    delivery, 123
Berthold-Bond, Annie, 38
Betacarotene, 116
Better Health Through Natural Healing
    (Trattler), 164
Biermann, June, 32
Biofeedback, 126
Bio-Integral Resource Center, 149
Biotin, abnormal need for, 12
Birth-control pills
    and breast-feeding, 135
Birth defects
    cause of, 5
    defined, 2
    incidence of, 2–4
    most common, 153–159
Birth Trap (Brackbill, Rice, and
    Young), 165
Birth weight. *See also* Birth weight, low
    and diabetes, 29
    and weight gain during pregnancy, 63
Birth weight, low
    and alcohol consumption, 76
    defined, 52
    financial problems and, 53, 56
    incidence of, 4
    smoking and, 81

stress and, 52–53
    underweight women and, 63
Birthing Normally (Peterson), 127
Birthmarks, 153
    incidence of, 3
Blood glucose level, testing, 31
Blood tests, 17–18
Blood type, incompatible, 119–120
    and Rho (D) immune globulin,
        119–120
Bonding, parent-child, 126–127
    and breast feeding, 132
Bower, John, 85
Brackbill, Yvonne, 123–24, 165
Brain development, and time of exposure
    to teratogens, 15
Breast-feeding, 131–36, 152
    benefits of, 132
    chemicals and, 132–36
    contraindications to, 137
    discontinuance of, 136
    drugs and, 132–136
    and Sudden Infant Death
        Syndrome, 142
Breech position
    and cesarean delivery, 125
    techniques to turn baby from, 127
Brewer, Gail S., 63
Brewer, Thomas, 32
*Brewer Medical Diet for Normal and High-
    Risk Pregnancy* (Brewer), 32
Brodeur, Paul, 98
Burns, Steven L., 57

Cadmium, 145
Caffeine, 77–78, 82
    breast-feeding and, 135
    smoking and, 82
Calcium, 59
    breast-feeding and, 132, 139
    sources of, 61
Cancer, 12. *See also* Anticancer drugs;
        Cancer, juvenile
    and prenatal exposure, 36–37
    susceptibility to, as birth defect, 2
Cancer, juvenile
    electromagnetic fields and, 146
    radiation exposure and, 94
Carbon monoxide, 83, 85–86
Carcinogens, 36–37. *See also* Cancer
        headings

Cassidy-Brinn, Ginny, 50–51, 103
Catalog of Teratogenic Agents (Shepard), 36, 74
Cataracts, 14, 71, 112
Cats, as toxoplasmosis carriers, 118–19
Cefalo, Robert, 24
Centers for Disease Control (CDC), 2, 4, 26, 27, 44, 58, 109
Central nervous system, and time of exposure to teratogens, 15
Cerebral palsy, 153–54
Cesarean section, 124–28
  breech position and, 125
  electronically monitored births and, 122
  failure to progress and, 125–26
  herpes virus transmission and, 115
  risks to mother, 124
  vaginal birth after, 124–25
Chemical Agents and Breast Milk (Lauwers and Woessner), 138–39
Chemical Exposures (Ashford and Miller), 87
Chemical Manufacturer's Association, 149
Chemicals. *See also* Drugs *headings;* Environmental toxicants; Pesticides
  avoiding exposure to, 152
  breast-feeding and, 132–36
  exposure of children to, 147–50
  in home, 84–87
  nontoxic alternatives to, 148–49
  sperm and, 40, 42–44
  in water supply, 88–89
Chicken pox, 107–8
Childbirth with Love (Lauersen), 50
Chorionic villus sampling (CVS), 19–20
Chromosomes, 6
  and gender-determination, 7
  and ionizing radiation, 94
  mutations of, 7–8
Cimetidine, 42
Clapp, James F., III, 101–2
Clean & Green (Berthold-Bond), 38
Cleft lip/palate, 154
  frequency of occurrence, 154
  vitamin supplements and, 59, 62
Club foot, 154
CMV. *See* Cytomegalovirus
Coach, during labor/delivery, 126–27
Cocaine, effects of, 79
Coffee consumption. *See* Caffeine
Cohen, Nancy Wainer, 128
Cold sores. *See* Herpes simplex

Collaborative Perinatal Project, 4, 126
Complete Guide to Mercury Toxicity from Dental Fillings (Taylor), 93
Computers, 98
Conception, 13–14
  and timing of intercourse, 16
Congenital varicella syndrome, 109
Consumer Products Safety Commission, 37
Contraceptives, oral, 25, 135
Corticosteroids, 69
Cosmic rays, 93–94
Coumadin, 72
Coumarin, 67
Counseling
  genetic, 11, 16–17
  for stress reduction, 56
Cross Currents (Becker), 98
Crystal, drinking from, 92
Currents of Death (Brodeur), 98
CVS. *See* Chorionic villus sampling
Cyclophosphamide, and breast-feeding, 134
Cyclosporine, and breast-feeding, 134
Cystic fibrosis, 11, 154–55
Cytomegalovirus (CMV), 110–11

Dadd, Debra Lynn, 38, 90
Dalmane, 123
Dance of Anger, The (Lerner), 56–57
Davis, Russell, 40
DDT, 42
Deafness, 112
Dean, Steve M., 96
Delivery. *See also* Cesarean section; Labor
  and breech position, 125
DES (diethylstilbestrol), 66
  effect of, on male offspring, 42
Diabetes mellitus, 25, 26, 28–32
  as birth defect, 2
  checklist of things to do, 30–32
  control of blood sugar in, 151
  gestational, 105–7
  juvenile (Type I), 29, 112
  risks associated with, 29–30
  self-care, 28–32
  Type I, 29, 112
  Type II, 29, 107
Diabetic Woman, The (Biermann, Toohey, and Jovanovic), 32
Diarrhea, and Sudden Infant Death Syndrome, 142

Diazepam, 70
Dibromochloropropane, 88
Diet. *See also* Nutrition
    and breast-feeding, 138
    reducing toxicity of foods through,
        90–91, 96
Diet for a Poisoned Planet (Steinman),
    90, 100
Diet pills, 71
Dieting. *See also* Diet; Nutrition
    before pregnancy, 63
    during pregnancy, 63
Digestive tract atresias, 155
Dilantin, 32, 42, 67
Dioxins, 43–44, 45
Diseases, infectious, 108–19
DNA (deoxyribonucleic acid), 6, 7
Dougherty, Robert C., 42
Doula, 126–27
Down syndrome, 5, 39, 155–56
    and alcohol consumption, 74
    blood test for, 17–18
    frequency of occurrence, 3, 156
    maternal age and, 15–16
    paternal age and, 15–16
Downer, Carol, 103
DPT immunizations, and Sudden Infant
        Death Syndrome, 142
Drugs, pharmaceutical, 45, 65–74
    and breast-feeding, 132–36, 138–39
    caffeine in, 78
    information sources, 73–74
    during labor, 123–124
    over-the-counter, 70–72
    passage across placenta, 65
    risks, 65
    solubility of, 133
    sperm and, 42
    stopping, 152
    teratogenic, 65–70
    and timing of consumption, 65, 66,
        67–68
Drugs, recreational, 75–82
    and breast-feeding, 137
    and semen, 41–42
    stopping, 152
Dysautonomia, familial, 9
Dystocia (failure to progress), 124,
    125–26

Ear development, and time of exposure to
    teratogens, 15

Easier Childbirth, An (Peterson),
    51, 128, 164
Echocardiograms, 18
Ectopic pregnancy, and smoking, 81
Edema, 64
Education, 50–51
Egg
    exposure to environmental hazards,
        13–14
    overripe, 15–16
Elavil, 68
Electric blankets, 96, 97
Electromagnetic radiation, 96–98
    effects on children, 146
    from high-power transmission lines, 98
    reducing exposure to, 97–98
Electronic monitoring of fetus,
    121–123, 125
    advantages and disadvantages of,
        121–122
    external, 121
    and herpes transmission, 122
    internal, 121, 122
England, Janice, 93
Environmental Protection Agency Radon
        Hotline, 96
Environmental toxicants, 1, 5, 12–16,
        83–100
    checklist of things to do, 38
    in home, 37–38
    infants and, 144–50
    occupational, 34–37
    to sperm, 40–45
    timing of exposure to, 14–15
Epidural analgesia, 125
Epilepsy, 32–33, 61–62. *See also*
        Anticonvulsant medications
Epilepsy Foundation of America, 33
Equal, 71
Ergotamine, and breast-feeding, 134
Erythromycin, and breast-
        feeding, 134
Ethnic groups, genetic diseases
        among, 10
Etretinate, 70
Everybody's Radiation Handbook (Dean), 96
Exercise, 101–4
    guidelines for, 103
    videotapes, 103–4
*Expectant Parent's Guide to Preventing a
        Cesarean Section, The* (Jones), 128
External version, 127

Eye development
  color, 8, 12
  and time of exposure to teratogens, 15

Failure to progress, 125–126
Family Genetic Sourcebook, The
      (Pierce), 164
Fathers, 39–45
  age of, 39
  alcohol consumption of, 76
  checklist of things to do, 44–46
  stress of, 56
Fava-ism, 8
Ferguson, Tom, 82
Fertility
  and environmental hazards, 40–41
  smoking and, 81
  sperm and, 41
Fetal alcohol syndrome, 75–76
Fetal monitoring, 115, 121–123, 125
Fifth disease (erythema infectiosum), 111
Financial problems, and low birth weight,
      53, 56
Fish
  mercury-accumulating, 91
  raw, avoiding, 61
Folic acid, 61
  and anticonvulsant medications, 62, 69
  aspirin and, 60
  birth-control pills and, 25
Food(s). *See also* Nutrition
  additives, and breast-feeding, 139
  cravings for, 64
  for newborn, 131–140
  organic, 100
Food and Drug Administration Total Diet
      Study, 59
Food chain, environmental toxins in, 88
For Our KIDS Sake (Garland), 148
For Tomorrow's Children, 26
Foresight, The Association for the
      Promotion of Preconceptual Care,
      23–24, 26
Formaldehyde, 86, 147–48
Formula-feeding, 136–37
  best choices for, 140
  nutrients lacking in, 136–37
Fragile X syndrome, 156
French program, 54–55
Friedman, Jan M., 39
Furniture, 148

Gantrisin, 68
Garland, Anne Witte, 100, 148
Garlic, 90
Gas fumes, 85–86, 149
Gastrointestinal defects, and maternal
      age, 15
Gastroschisis, 156
Genetic counseling, 11, 16–17
Genetic inheritance, 5, 6, 7
  and birth defects, 5–6
  dominant traits in, 8–9
  multiple genes, diseases based upon,
      11–12
  mutations and, 8–9, 11
  recessive traits in, 9–11
Genital herpes. *See* Herpes simplex
Genitalia, development of, and time of
      exposure to teratogens, 15
German measles (rubella), 14, 112–13
  birth defects due to, 112
  immunization against, 112, 113
  test for immunity, 25, 112
Getting the Love You Want (Hendrix), 57
Ginger, 73–74
Glucose, control of, 105–6
Gofman, John W., 95
Good Birth, A Safe Birth, A (Korte and
      Scaer), 165
Greenfield, Ellen J., 86
*Guide to Hazardous Products Around the
      Home* (HHWP), 86–87

Haertel, Lois, 89
Hair dryers, 97
Having Your Baby When Others Say No!
      (Nugent), 164–165
Healing Yourself During Pregnancy
      (Gardner), 164
Healthy House, The (Bower), 86
Heart defects/diseases, 12,
      112, 156
  echocardiogram testing for, 18
  incidence of, 3
  rubella and, 14
Hemophilia, 5
Hendrix, Harville, 57
Henshaw, Denis, 146
Heparin, 73
Hepatitis B, 113–14
  testing for, 113–14
Heroin, effects of, 79–80

Herpes simplex, 114–117
    transmission to infant, 115
Herpes zoster, 108–9
Hip, congenitally dislocated, 154
Hispanics, 4
    and Sudden Infant Death
        Syndrome, 141
HIV (human immunodeficiency virus),
        27–28
    test for, 28
Home, toxicants in. *See* Indoor pollution
Homeopathic remedies, 73
Hornstein, Francie, 103
Hospitals, position on fetal
        monitoring, 122
Hotlines, 160–63
House Dangerous (Greenfield), 86
How to Survive Unbearable Stress
        (Burns), 57
Huggins, Hal A., 93
Human chorionic gonadotropin, 17–18
Hydrocephalus, 10, 156
Hypercholestrolemia, familial, 11
Hypertension, 12
Hypnosis
    and premature labor, 54
    self-, 126
Hypoglycemia, 31
Hypoglycemic drugs, oral, and birth
        defects, 31
Hypospadias, 71, 156–157

Ibuprofen, 72
Immune suppressive agents, and breast-
        feeding, 134
Immune system
    of infant, and breast-feeding, 134
    and radiation, 94
Immunizations, and Sudden Infant Death
        Syndrome, 142, 143
Indoor pollution, 36–37
    air, 84–87
    exposure of children to, 147–50
    and Sudden Infant Death
        Syndrome, 142
Infant Formula Act, 137
Infectious diseases. *See* Diseases,
        infectious
Insulin levels, 106
International Cesarean Awareness
        Network, 127

International Lactation Consultants
        Association (ILCA), 138
Intravenous drip, during labor, 125
Iron, in diet, 59
Isoniazid, and breast-feeding, 134
It's All in Your Head (Huggins), 93

Jacobson, Michael P., 100
Jampolsky, Gerald, 56
"Jane Fonda's New Pregnancy Workout"
        (videotape), 104
Japanese, 143
Jews, 9, 159
Jones, Carl, 128, 165
Jovanovic, Lois, 32

Kamen, Betty, 63, 139
Kamen, Si, 63
"Kathy Smith's Pregnancy Workout"
        (videotape), 104
Kelley-Buchanan, Christine, 74
Kelp, 90, 96
Kennell, John, 126
Ketoacidosis, 29
Ketoprofen, 69
Kitzinger, Sheila, 51
Klaus, Marshall, 126
Koehler, Nan, 128
Korte, Diana, 165
Kunin, Richard, 116

La Leche League, 138
Labels, reading, 148
Labor
    failure to progress, 125–26
    walking around during, 122, 125
Lactation consultants, 138
Lactose intolerance, 157
Lamache, Alexandre, 75
Landfills, 92
Lauerson, Niels, 50
Lauwers, Judith, 138–39
Lead, 90, 95
    in air, 82
    blood test for, 25, 91, 133–34, 144–45
    in body, 25, 45, 91
    breast-feeding and, 133–34
    household sources of, 91
    protecting child from, 144–46

school performance and, 144–45
testing environment for, 92, 145
in water supply, 87–88
Learning disabilities, 4, 144–45
Lefferts, Lisa Y., 100
Lerner, Harriet Goldhor, 56–57
Lesch-Nyhan syndrome, 39
Leukemia, childhood, 43, 44
and electromagnetism, 98
and pesticides, 99
Levodopa, and breast-feeding, 134
Librium, 123
Lightbox, effects of, 98
Limb development, and time of exposure
to teratogens, 15
Linolenic acid, in formula, 137, 140
Lithium, 67
and breast-feeding, 134
Liver diseases, chronic, and hepatitis B,
113, 114
Love Is Letting Go of Fear (Jampolsky), 56
LSD, 78, 79

Macler, Bruce, 89
Magnesium, in diet, 59
March of Dimes, 2, 17, 44, 45, 50
Marfan syndrome, 39
Marijuana, 45, 78–79
effects of, 79
sperm and, 41–42
Maternal Serum Alpha-fetoprotein
(MSAFP), 17–18
Meat, rare or raw, avoiding, 61, 118
Medications. *See* Drugs, pharmaceutical
Meditation, 126
Mega-Nutrition for Women (Kunin), 116
Mehl, Lewis E., 53–54
Mental disorders, incidence of, 4
Mercury, 85, 90, 145
in body, 45, 133–34
breast-feeding and, 133–34
sources of, 91
in water supply, 88
Methadone, effects of, 79–80
Methotrexate, 68
Methylmercury, 88
Metronidazole, and breast-feeding, 134
Migraine medication, and breast-
feeding, 134
Miller, Claudia S., 87
Mineral deficiencies, 59–61

Mineral supplements, 60–61, 82, 152
Monitoring. *See also* Electronic monitoring
of fetus
by nurses, 121–122
Moos, Merry-K., 24
Morning sickness, 73, 74
Motrin, 71–72
Mott, Lawrie, 100
Moxibustion, correcting breech position
with, 127
Muscular dystrophy, 157

Naprosyn, 69
National Academy of Science, 63
National Information Service (NIS), 45
National Institutes of Health, 124
National Pesticide Telecommunications
Network, 100
Native Americans, infant mortality, 4
Natural Choices, 149–50
Needleman, Herbert L., 87
Nervous system, development of, 13–14.
See also Neural tube defects
Neural tube defects, 43. *See also*
Anencephaly; Spina bifida
ethnic group and, 10
and folic acid deficiency, 26, 59
incidence of, 59
MSAFP testing for, 17
surgery during pregnancy and, 50
and time of exposure to teratogens, 15
vitamin supplements and, 58–59
zinc and, 59
Neuroblatoma, and pesticides, 99
Nicotine. *See* Smoking
Niemann-Pick disease, 9
Nighttime Parenting (Sears), 142–43
Nipples, stimulating, during labor, 127
*No-Nag, No-Guilt, Do It Your Own Way
Guide to Quitting Smoking, The*
(Ferguson), 82
Nontoxic, Natural, & Earthwise (Dadd),
38, 90
Nontoxic alternatives, using, 148–49
Nontoxic Baby, The (Natural Choices),
149–50
NutraSweet, 71
Nutrition, 44–45, 58–64, 151. *See
also* Diet checklist, 61–63
individual differences in
requirements, 59
Recommended Dietary Allowance, 59

Nutritional counseling, 62
Nutritional deficiencies
    and birth defects, 58–63
    explanations for, 59–62
    symptoms, 59

Obstetricians, checking cesarean rates
    of, 126
Occupational hazards, 34–38. *See also*
    Chemicals; Environmental toxins;
    Indoor pollution; Teratogens
    checking, 45
    sperm and, 42–44
O'Connor, Egan, 95
Omega-3 fatty acid, 136
Omphalocele, 157
Onions, 90
Open Season (Cohen), 128
Orudis, 69
Oxytocin
    effect of, on infant, 126
    intravenous, 125–26
    stress and, 125

Painkillers, and breast-feeding, 135–36
Paints, 85
    lead in, 144, 145
Palate development, 15. *See also* Cleft
    lip/palate
Papiernik, Emile, 54–55
Parkinson's disease medication, and
    breast-feeding, 134
Parvovirus B19, 111
PCBs (polychlorinated biphenyls), 42
Peace of Mind During Pregnancy (Kelley-
    Buchanan), 74
Perchloroethylene, 88
    and breast-feeding, 133
Pesticide Alert (Mott and Snyder), 100
Pesticides, 99–100
    blood test for, 25
    breast-feeding and, 139
    exposure of children to, 147, 148
    natural, 100
    reducing exposure to, 99–100
    sperm and, 40
    washing off food, 100
Peterson, Gayle, 51, 127, 128, 164
Phenylketonuria (PKU), 11, 71, 157–58
Phenylpropanolamine, 72

Phenytoin, 10, 32, 42
Physician's Desk Reference, 74
Pierce, Benjamin A., 164
Pitocin, 125
PKU. *See* Phenylketonuria
Placenta previa, and smoking, 81
Placental separation, 79
Plumbing, as source of lead, 88, 90
Poisoning Our Children (Sokol), 150
Polio immunizations, and Sudden Infant
    Death Syndrome, 142
Pollutants. *See* Environmental toxicants
Polydactyly, 71, 158
Pottery, testing for lead, 92
Preconception care, 23–26
    checklist of things to do, 24–26
Preconceptual Health Appraisal, 24
Pregnancy and Childbirth (Hotchner), 50
Premature delivery
    defined, 52
    French model of perinatal intervention,
        54–55
    prevention of, 54
    stress and, 52–53
Prenatal care, 49–51. *See also*
        Preconception care
    benefits of, 49
    checklist of things to do, 50–51
Prenatal testing, 16–20
Preventive medicine, 23
Primidone, and breast-feeding, 134
Progestins, 66
Prolactin, 132
Prolactin suppressant, and breast-
    feeding, 134
Proloprim, and breast-feeding, 134
Psoriasis remedy, and breast-feeding, 134
Pyloric stenosis, 158

Rachel (Remote Access Chemical Hazards
    Electronic Library), 36
Radiation, 1, 89
    contamination of water supply by, 89
    exposure of parent to, 13
    ionizing, 93–96, 146
    limiting exposure to, 95
    male fertility and, 45
    nonionizing (*see* Electromagnetic
        radiation)
    sperm and, 44
Radiology drugs, and breast-feeding, 136

Radium, in water supply, 89
Radon, 89, 93–95
  testing for, 95–96
  in water supply, 89
Reducing Exposure to Lead in Older Homes
    (Roberts), 146
Relaxation during labor, 126
  intravenous oxytoxin and, 125–26
Research reports, medical, obtaining, 74
Retinoblastoma, 11
Rice, June, 165
Risk factors, 4–5
Roberts, John R., 145, 146
Robinson, Margaret, 60
Rothman, Cappy, 40–41
Rubella. *See* German measles

Saccharine, 71
Safe Drinking Water and Toxic
    Enforcement Act (1986), 34–35, 43
Safe Food (Jacobson, Lefferts, and
    Garland), 100
Salt, in diet, 60, 61
Samuels, Michael, 50
Samuels, Nancy, 50
Savitz, David, 146
Scaer, Roberta, 165
Sears, William, 142–43
Seaweed, 90, 96
Sedatives, 70
Septra, 68
Sexually transmitted diseases, 28
Shakespeare, William, 52
Shepard, Thomas H., 36, 74
Shingles, 108–9
Sickle-cell anemia. *See* Anemia,
    sickle-cell
SIDS. *See* Sudden Infant Death Syndrome
SIDS Alliance, 143
Silver (amalgam) fillings, 91, 92–93
Sleep patterns, shared, and SIDS, 142–43
Smoking, 5, 12, 25, 45, 52, 80–82, 85–86
  and breast-feeding, 135
  effects on children, 147
  sperm and, 41
  stopping, 81–82, 152
Snyder, Karen, 100
Sokol, Nancy, 150
Special Supplemental Food Program for
    Women, Infants, and Children
    (WIC), 62

Sperm
  environmental influences on, 13–14,
    40–45
  production of, 13–14
Sperm banks, 45
Spina bifida, 44, 158–59
  alcohol consumption and, 75
  folic acid and, 62
  frequency of occurrence, 3, 158
  MSAFP testing for, 17
  ultrasound testing for, 18
  vitamin supplements and, 58–59
Steinman, David, 90, 100
Stimulants, and breast-feeding, 134
Stress, emotional, 16, 52–54
  direct and indirect effects, 52–53
  of fathers, 56
  oxytocin and, 125
  reduction of, 53–54, 55–57, 82
  during second trimester, 53
Sudden Infant Death Syndrome (SIDS),
    79, 141–43
  and breast-feeding, 132
  risk factors, 141–42, 143
  smoking and, 81
Sulfa drugs, 68
  and breast-feeding, 134–35
Support, social, 56
Support during labor, 126–27
Surgery during pregnancy. *See also*
    Cesarean section
  and neural tube defects, 50
Syphilis, 117–18

Tagamet, 42
Taylor, Joyal, 93
Tay-Sachs Disease, 8, 9, 159
  blood test for, 17
  frequency of occurrence, 159
  genetic counseling and, 11
Tea consumption, 77–78
Tegison, 70
  and breast-feeding, 134
Teratogens, 34–35. *See also* Environmental
    toxicants; Drugs *headings;* Indoor
    pollution; Occupational hazards
  checklist of things to do, 36–37
  sperm and, 40–45
Testing, prenatal, 16–20
Testosterone, 66
Thalassemia, 10

Thalidomide, 1, 41
Tinidazole, and breast-feeding, 134
Toohey, Barbara, 32
Tooth development, and time of exposure
    to teratogens, 15
Total Nutrition During Pregnancy (Kamen
    and Kamen), 63
Total Nutrition for Breast-Feeding Mothers
    (Kamen), 139–40
Toxoplasmosis, 118–19
Tranquilizers
    and breast-feeding, 134
    during labor/delivery, 123
Trattler, Ross, 164
Trichloroethane, 88
Trichloroethylene, 88
Tridione, 32
Trimethadione, 32, 66
Trimethoprim, and breast-feeding, 134
Tris, 42
Trisodium phosphate (TSP), washing
    with, 92, 146
Tylenol, 70–71

Ulcer drugs, 42
Ulene, Art, 103
Ultrasound, described, 18
Underweight women, 63, 64
U.S. Department of
    Education, 4

Vaccines, 71. *See also* Immunization
Vaginal birth after cesarean (VBAC),
    124–25
Valium, 65, 70, 122
Valproic acid, 67
Varicella. *See* Chicken pox
Varicella syndrome, congenital, 109
Varicella-zoster immune globulin
    (VZIG), 109
Video display terminals (VDTs),
    96–97, 98
Vinyl chloride, 43
Viral infections, 108–17
Visualization for an Easier Childbirth (Jones),
    128

Vitamin supplements, 25, 60–61, 82, 152
    excessive, avoiding, 62
    neural tube defects and, 58–59
Vomiting, in infant, and Sudden Infant
    Death Syndrome, 142

Walking around during labor, 122, 125
Warfarin, 67, 72
Washington Toxics Coalition, 149
Waste dumps, toxic, 91–92, 93
Water supply
    polluted, 87–89
    tap versus bottled, 90
    testing, 89–90
Weed, Susan, 63
Weight gain during pregnancy, 63–64
Well Pregnancy Book (Samuels and
    Samuels), 50
Wertheimer, Nancy, 96, 146
What Every Pregnant Woman Should Know
    (Brewer), 63
What to Expect When You're Expecting
    (Eisenberg), 51
*Wise-Woman Herbal for the Childbearing
    Year* (Weed), 63
Withdrawal symptoms, in infants,
    78, 79–80
Woessner, Candace, 138–39
Woman-Centered Pregnancy and Birth
    (Cassidy-Brinn, Hornstein, and
    Downer), 51, 103
Work environment. *See* Indoor pollution;
    Occupational hazards
Wynn, Arthur and Margaret, 23

X rays, 26, 94, 95
X rays: Health Effects of Common Exams
    (Gofman and O'Connor), 95

Yoga, 78
Young, Diony, 165

Zinc
    aspirin and, 60
    deficiency of, 58
    in diet, 59, 116